The Self-Directed Learner in Medical Education

The Three Pillar Model for developing self-directedness

JENNY GAVRIEL

Programme Director, Milton Keynes GP Specialty
Training Programme
Affiliate Lecturer, Post Graduate Certificate in
Clinical Education, Health Education Thames Valley
with Oxford Brookes University
Tutor, Post Graduate Certificate of Education
University of Buckingham

Radcliffe Publishing
London • New York

Radcliffe Publishing Ltd
St Mark's House
Shepherdess Walk
London N1 7BQ
United Kingdom

www.radcliffehealth.com

British Library Cataloguing in Publication Data

A catalogue record for this book is available from the British Library.

ISBN-13: 978 190936 844 6

The paper used for the text pages of this book is FSC® certified. FSC (The Forest Stewardship Council®) is an international network to promote responsible management of the world's forests.

Typeset by Darkriver Design, Auckland, New Zealand
Manufacturing managed by 21six

Contents

Preface

The development of self-directedness is an educational conundrum that transcends medical education. My time in education with children and adults in schools and in medical education has revealed a common complaint: educators at every stage want their learners to take more responsibility and more initiative in their learning. It is a common frustration that many learners are passive in their educational role and although self-directedness is often seen as a purely adult learning concept, similar concerns are expressed in school staff rooms across the country. This book is based on the reality that we cannot assume learners will become self-directed as they mature. I have seen teenagers whose ability and motivation in directing their own learning far outstrips that of some adult learners, both in teaching and in medical education. We need to build a learning and working environment that supports and nurtures self-directedness.

As I broadened my educational experience and extended my reading in educational literature and research I began to realise that there were strategies out there to help develop self-directedness. It became apparent that this was not something that could be achieved through just one area of research. Writing this book has been a tremendous learning opportunity for me, and I hope you will find it as useful as I have. You should find a combination of new ideas and new perspectives to old ideas, as well as new knowledge; this is the opportunity to revisit prior knowledge with a different hat on. There is a lot of information within these pages: the Three Pillar Model provides an overarching structure for the book, but each subsequent chapter has been researched from specific areas. Throughout each chapter I have tried to tread the line between theory and practical, to find the balance between evidence-based education and usefulness at the front line.

I have attempted to write this book in such a way that recognises and respects the skills that you bring to your educational practice. Much of education is context specific and individualistically driven so the techniques described here are intended to become useful additions to your toolkit. Your skills and experience are needed to know when and how to deploy them. This is not an easy task, but your current expertise combined with this book will provide you with the skills and support to meet this challenge.

Though I hope you will find the style of writing accessible and the structure clear, this is not a book that you will pick up and read cover to cover in a few days. Take your time over it and give yourself the opportunity to reflect on your strengths and areas for development. I am probably biased, but I do think everything in this book is useful; the educators' toolkit needs to be as large and diverse as possible. This is especially the case when looking to develop a complex skill like self-directedness. Of course you cannot be expected to do everything. Education is a hard task master: there is always more that can be done; a better or different way to do things; new ideas to be trialled. There are so many ideas in this book that it can at first glance seem daunting. You have to accept from the start that you cannot attempt all of these ideas at once. Instead you should read through and prioritise according to your own needs, your learner and your context. Try out a few ideas and let them bed in, then return to look through the model again and see if there is something else to try. Take a step-wise approach to constructing an environment and improving your skills to develop self-directed learners.

Having said all of this, the content of this book doesn't represent everything. Not even close. There is so much more out there and I hope that if you find something of particular interest you will also find the references you need to follow up in greater depth. I repeatedly had to restrain myself and cease typing mid-flow to prevent myself going too far with each specific point. I am (obviously) passionate about education and the writing of this book has been an edifying experience for me. Pulling together the various and diverse ideas from different areas of research has been both useful and satisfying. I hope you gain as much as I have and that you find enough breadth and depth to meet your specific needs.

And one last thing: I have mistyped self-directed as elfs-directed so many times in writing this book that I am beginning to suspect the elves may actually be up to something.

Jenny Gavriel
January 2015

About the author

Jenny Gavriel initially qualified as a secondary school teacher in science and chemistry from the Institute of Education, London following completion of her degree in biochemistry with management from Imperial College London. She took her education studies further during her time in the classroom, gaining a Masters in Education from Oxford Brookes University. She also found time to produce resource sets for use by teachers which were published and sold nationally. After a number of years of teaching, during which time she held posts in curriculum planning, mentoring and pastoral management, her career shifted focus from educating children to educating adults. She now sits on the line between the two worlds: school education and medical education, giving her a broad view of the direction of education in general.

As Programme Director for GP Specialty Training in Milton Keynes, Jenny has frontline contact with medical learners, while she maintains an academic focus as an Affiliate Lecturer on the Post Graduate Certificate in Clinical Education for Health Education Thames Valley. She retains contact with education in the school environment as a Tutor for trainee teachers with the University of Buckingham.

Jenny has published articles in the *British Journal of General Practice* and *Education for Primary Care* and writes regular 'Teaching Tips' in *Education for Primary Care* which draws on her expertise in both school-based education and medical education.

Further details regarding Jenny's work can be found at www.GavrielMedEd.com.

List of figures

List of tables

CHAPTER 1

A model for self-directedness

'We've got this saying, "performance by the aggregation of marginal gains". It means taking the 1% from everything you do; finding a 1% margin for improvement in everything you do.'[1]

Sir David Brailsford

INTRODUCTION

Educating others is fundamental to individual and societal improvement; it has to rank as one of the most, if not the most, important of trades. To paraphrase Dewey,[2] while DNA provides the mechanism for the continuation of biology, education is the mechanism for the continuation of society. We, as a human race, have reached our advanced stage of societal development because educators at all stages of learning have provided the mechanism for society to improve and achieve. Yet, still, we are not perfect and so the next generation of educators (that's us) steps forward to use our expertise to develop the knowledge, skills and attitudes that enable our learners to move medicine and healthcare forwards.

With the importance of the role of the educator in mind, when we become educators we accept a responsibility to strive for excellence. Though medical education is often altruistic in nature, we must constantly seek to improve our practice and in doing so improve the outcomes for our learners individually and as part of a forward-moving community. The community we are educating in is not the one in which our learners will be working. In reality the healthcare community is constantly evolving and will become increasingly unrecognisable to those who worked in healthcare 50 years ago and difficult to imagine for those of us here today. Health Education England predicts 'A significant part of the workforce in 2030 will find themselves working flexibly across specialisms and care settings in roles and places of work largely unfamiliar to the workforce today.[3] [(p. 6)] Most of us can probably see this coming, but predicting what the outcome will really look like in the final draft is beyond my powers.

This constant progression is not unique to healthcare and many organisations today, the National Health Service (NHS) included, strive to be 'learning organisa-tions'. These are organisations that seek to facilitate the learning of their employees and are open and willing to learn and change at an organisational level.

It is against this background that we begin to see the importance of the self-directed learner. We work in a community where standing still is going backwards; therefore we need workers with a desire to learn and the ability to do so without direct supervision. As educators we cannot simply assume that self-directed learning is pre-programmed into all learners; instead we must put in place mechanisms to develop the skills, motivations and self-belief for our learners to become self-directed both in the immediate learning experience and throughout the rest of their career.

Self-directed learning is perhaps the Holy Grail of adult learning and for good reason. Within this seemingly simple phrase lies the battleground for the frus-trations of both educator and learner as they work through the difficulties of an unequal and sometimes intense partnership. The busy educator needs to guide the learner successfully through their learning with the knowledge that the best long-term outcome is a self-directed learner. Working against this is the knowledge that, in the short term, it is quicker and easier to tell them the answer. Meanwhile, the busy learner is under pressure from all sides and wants the answer handed to them with a minimum of fuss. It seems to me, as someone who has taught teenagers as well as adults, that the latter tend to revert to the former when they take on the 'learner' label. Think about the last time you went on a course. What did you look at when you received the schedule for the day? You probably glanced down the lec-tures or workshops, but did your eye linger longer on the timings of the breaks? Did you find yourself thinking about what might be laid on for lunch given the chosen venue? Did you look at the end time and wonder if you could get home earlier than usual? If not, congratulations; you are truly a very focused individual, but you are the exception. Keeping in mind that even the best of us are not always as focused as we perhaps should be will help dissipate the mounting frustrations of working with adult learners who seem to have a Peter Pan approach to learning and just will not act like adults.

'Self-directed learning' has been circulating as a buzz phrase in education for many decades now. The past few decades have seen increasing interest in the idea of learning organisations, career-long professional development and lifelong edu-cation. Accreditations such as 'Investors in People' are evidence of the focus on continual development for many businesses. As part of this progress the self-directed movement has grown and now finds itself firmly embedded in many adult learning contexts. So it seems self-directed learning is here to stay as one of the most important aspects, if not the most important, of adult education. After all, to steal from an old proverb: 'You can lead a horse to water, but you can't make it drink.' If we want our learner to continue drinking from the educational well (sorry, may have taken the old adage a step too far there) after their formal education, we must find a way to instil in them a high level of self-directedness. Obvious, I think, yes. Easy, most definitely, no. After many decades of work the magic bullet to create self-directedness continues to elude researchers in adult education. Most probably because there is no magic bullet, no quick fix. Sorry. The development of self-directedness is a complex beast. Individual psyches, varying intellects and personal motivations are all bundled up to create our learners, making each and every one of them unique and therefore the mechanism to promote self-directedness in them equally unique.

THE THREE PILLAR MODEL OF SELF-DIRECTEDNESS

If self-directedness is our cake, the raw ingredient is our learner. As adult educators we have to 'bake' our learner to make them self-directed, and in order to do this we need a recipe. OK, so I may be forcing the analogy somewhat but stick with it. In this chapter we will construct a model that provides us with a recipe, a system for considering what we need to put into place to develop self-directed learners.

This model is built upon research from many relevant fields combined with half a cup of experience and a pinch of common sense (definitely pushing the analogy now, sorry). It is fundamentally based upon the 'aggregation of marginal gains': any single action or change in methodology is unlikely to have a significant impact upon the learner's self-directedness, but taken together the right combination of factors will add up to substantial change.

In this model, the ultimate aim – self-directedness – is a block held up by three pillars, each of which is necessary for successful self-directedness (*see* Figure 1.1).

- Skills – learners must have the skills necessary to complete the learning process and insight into their own strengths and weaknesses in relation to these skills.
- Motivation – learners need motivating in order to complete the tasks associated with their formal learning; they also need to develop an understanding of their own personal motivations to ensure they can continue to be self-directed in future situations.
- Self-belief – learners have to believe that they are capable of completing the task successfully.

Each of these pillars is necessary to support the characteristic of self-directedness; remove one of the pillars and self-directedness will fall down. We will discuss each of these pillars in more detail soon, but first we will look more closely at how the self-directedness block is supported by the three pillars.

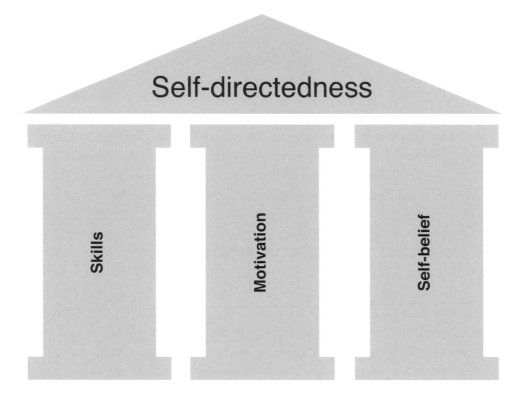

FIGURE 1.1 A three-pillar model of self-directedness

Self-directedness

The fundamental concept of the three pillar structure is that the learner will need each of these pillars in place if they are to successfully become self-directed. If one (or two) is missing they are unlikely to develop a self-directed approach to their learning.

Without the Skills Pillar

If the learner has the motivation and a high level of belief that they are capable of completing the task but lacks the skills required to successfully negotiate the learning process, they will probably make an attempt at the task. However, without the skills they are likely to fail, or at least only succeed at a superficial level; this will impact upon their self-belief and likely damage internal motivating factors.

Without the Motivation Pillar

If the learner has the skills combined with a high level of self-belief but lacks the motivational factors, they will be unlikely to attempt the task. For some learners (and some tasks) the task itself, and the belief that they are capable of doing it, may be enough to provide motivation. However, this needs to be considered by either the educator or the learner when undertaking a task.

Without the Self-belief Pillar

If the learner has the learning skills and the motivation but a low level of self-belief they will not believe they can successfully complete the task. They will either make no attempt at the task or will attempt it with little enthusiasm, thus reducing their chances of successful or effective completion. The consequence of the latter outcome is further damage to their level of self-belief, preventing attempts at future tasks and entering the learner into a negative cycle: low self-belief, leading to inhibited effort and enthusiasm, followed by failure, causing a further drop in their level of self-belief.

It is the combination of all three pillars that has the strength to support self-directedness. If we can put in place suitable mechanisms to develop the necessary skills, motivation and self-belief in our learners, we can build up each of the three pillars. In the following chapters we will look for metaphorical bricks that could be used to build each pillar in our model. These are the things educators can do to teach learning skills, improve motivation and develop self-belief. First, though, we will look in further detail at the structure of each of the pillars. We will use some well-known and well-regarded theoretical models to provide us with a number of categories in each pillar to help organise our thoughts about each aspect of self-directedness.

THE SKILLS PILLAR

In order for our learners to become truly self-directed in their learning we must provide them with the skills to learn from experience. Self-directed learning should be more than simply selecting a course from the limited few available or affordable or within the appropriate timescale for their next performance review. It should be experiential in nature and part of a continual process of learning, but this requires an understanding of the experiential learning process. Therefore, we must identify and help the learner develop an implicit and explicit understanding of their learning. In childhood education the learner is led through the learning process, being very much guided and supported by their teacher, and as learners mature, their ability to take over this process to varying degrees will develop. If we are to expect self-directedness from our adult learners, it is only fair we ensure they have the necessary skills to negotiate the learning process. Their subsequent workplace learning may be entirely self-directed with learners negotiating the learning process independently. There are some workplaces where it is common practice for a 'light touch' mentoring process, but often individual development is still self-sought. In formal education settings the learning process tends to be quite organised and carefully structured to build upon prior knowledge. Learning in the workplace, however, is likely to be far less stepwise than many learning cycles would suggest. The skilled learner will manage to meet each point on the cycle without having to strictly adhere to the prescribed stages of learning. By providing the learner with learning skills during the more formalised learning processes we give them the ability to cope in an often chaotic workplace (at least it is in my world) where they may have little to no formal support.

It is important to emphasise that the skills we are talking about in this pillar are the skills necessary to learn; that is, the knowledge and insight that a learner must develop to be able to guide themselves through the learning process. This pillar does not relate to the skills that the learner may need to acquire in order to meet learning objectives, competences or curriculum statements. One of the (many) challenges for educators is to ensure adequate focus on learning skills and not get caught up entirely in the content of the learning. It is tempting, particularly when there is a curriculum and a deadline involved, to focus on the knowledge and skills required to meet these objectives. If, however, we intend to develop self-directed learners, their understanding of the learning process is an essential consideration during all interactions.

Experiential learning

Experiential learning put in its simplest form is the idea that we learn from experience. Not exactly rocket science to the modern educator. It has become firmly embedded in the foundations of all education but particularly in adult education. Though it can be argued that all ages are constantly learning from experience (yesterday my two-year-old daughter learned that a goat 'baas' like a sheep because she heard it at the farm), for the purposes of this book we will obviously focus on adult education.

Cognitively based learning cycles are relatively abstract in nature; they are embedded in the internal, mental activity involved in the learning process. Behavioural models provide less room for conscious thought, being based within subconscious behaviours, with the stimulus rather than the individual determining the behaviour. Experiential learning combines cognitive with behavioural within a broader, more holistic, reality-driven setting. The importance of experiential learning for adult education has been emphasised repeatedly, not least by Knowles[4] who included the role of experience as the second of his four assumptions of adult learning. It is logical, therefore, to use experiential learning as a mechanism for identifying the learning skills necessary for self-directed learning. As such, the structure of the Skills Pillar in our model of self-directedness will be based on experiential learning.

Experiential learning has been popularised by Kolb's learning cycle,[5] but actually the basis for this approach to learning lies much earlier in educational research. Kolb's work drew heavily upon previous work on experiential learning by both Dewey and Lewin.

Dewey[2] was acutely aware that an individual's learning takes place within a wider context and that there has to be an interactive, social element to learning. His research explored the impact of setting learning opportunities into real life contexts. He believed teaching should focus on experience not didactic lecturing or asking learners to plough through textbooks (we'll ignore the irony of this being a textbook). His fundamental philosophy was that learning is most effective when it is combined with genuine experience. This seems, to me at least, to be fairly obvious, but in the early 1900s the traditional view of learning was strongly held and Dewey was proposing fairly radical changes to the teaching methods of the time.

> An experience, a very humble experience, is capable of generating and carrying any amount of theory (or intellectual content), but a theory apart from an experience cannot be definitely grasped even as theory. It tends to become a mere verbal formula, a set of catchwords used to render thinking, or genuine theorising, unnecessary and impossible.[2 (p. 80)]

There is nothing that an educational writer likes more than a good cycle. Reflective cycles, action research cycles, educational cycles, learning cycles, we will see so many of them throughout this book we risk dizziness and nausea. Nonetheless, here we go: Dewey's work (as illustrated by Kolb) laid some very solid foundations for the experiential learning movement (*see* Figure 1.2). What begins to emerge is a key skill for all: controlling the initial reactive impulse to allow time for observations, reflections and the cognitive collation of new information.

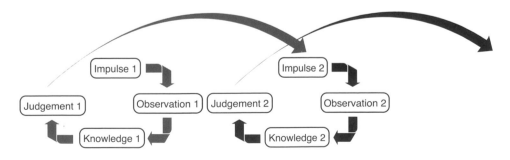

FIGURE 1.2 Dewey's Experiential Learning Cycle (as illustrated by Kolb)

One of the other key influencers of the experiential learning movement was Lewin. Kolb[5] discussed the relevance of Lewin's work in the introduction to his Experiential Learning Cycle. Lewin based much of his work around action research cycles (we will come to these in Chapter 5). He felt that much of the ineffectiveness of individual and organisational behaviour could be traced to an imbalance between action and observation. We've all met people at each of these extremes – those who spend so much time observing they never get anything done and those who rush headlong into action and fall over themselves. He borrowed the idea of feedback loops from electrical engineering and pieced it together with his research into learning. The outcome was a cycle which provides a goal-orientated, reflective action approach to learning; *see* Figure 1.3.

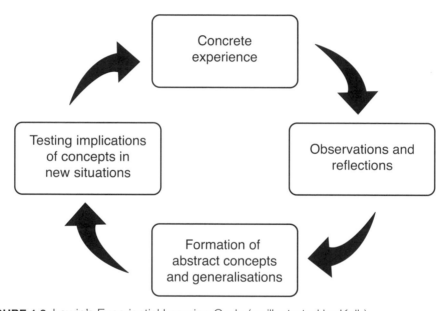

FIGURE 1.3 Lewin's Experiential Learning Cycle (as illustrated by Kolb)

The learning process is initiated by some form of practical experience. The following stages of reflection on the experience, absorption of the details and subsequent examination of the new information complete the cycle to feed back into another concrete experience when the new information is put into action.

Kolb's Experiential Learning Cycle[5]

Like many things in educational research, Kolb's learning cycle was built upon the work of researchers, like the aforementioned Dewey and Lewin and also Piaget, who is often seen as a founding father of experiential learning and constructivism. Using their ideas as a foundation, Kolb discussed the nature of learning and identified a continuum of learning. He suggested that learning is not a single thing that takes place in allocated places of learning. Instead he identified a continuum from specific performances, to learning, to long-term development (*see* Figure 1.4).

> Typically, an immediate reaction to a limited situation or problem is not thought of as learning but as performance. Similarly at the other extreme, we do not commonly think of long-term adaptations to one's total life situation as learning but as development. Yet performance, learning and development, viewed from the perspective of experiential learning theory, form a continuum of adaptive postures to the environment, varying only in their degree of extension in time and space. Performance is limited to short term adaptations to immediate circumstance, learning encompasses somewhat longer term mastery of generic classes of situations and development encompasses lifelong adaptation to one's total life situation.[5 (p. 34)]

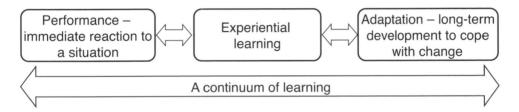

FIGURE 1.4 Kolb's continuum of learning

Brookfield[6] divided experiential learning into two realms. First, there is the learning taking place from direct participation in life's events; the immediate learning from 'that went well/that went badly' thought processes that determine how we will deal with a repeat of a particular experience in the future. These instantaneous reflections on performance under a particular circumstance are one type of experiential learning. The alternative is the learning undertaken by students who are taught in more formal environments but provided with appropriate activities from which to gain experience. These (usually) more structured and prescribed learning experiences form the second realm of experiential learning. If we consider Brookfield's realms of experiential learning in the context of Kolb's continuum of learning, we can see that the two realms are really part of the same continuum rather than two separate ideas. The instantaneous reflections on performance are one end of Kolb's continuum while the formal learning realm lies in the middle of the continuum. In combination, over a long time period, these two realms will lead to the development of the individual in a broader manner. Thus experiential learning can be found at the heart of the whole continuum of learning, and it becomes apparent that the learning process in each of these circumstances must have similarities that can be drawn together. Experiential learning is not just for workplace reflections, it allows us to scrutinise learning in all situations: formal, informal, short term, long term, teacher led or learner led.

Kolb's learning cycle (*see* Figure 1.5) is firmly rooted in experiential learning and is constructed from four stages of the learning process, very similar to those proposed by Lewin. Kolb used these four stages to identify and classify the differing sets of abilities needed for each stage:

● concrete experience abilities: learners 'must be able to involve themselves fully, openly and without bias in new experiences'

● reflective observation abilities: learners 'must be able to reflect on and observe their experiences from many perspectives'

● abstract conceptualisation abilities: learners 'must be able to create concepts that integrate their observations into logically sound theory'

● active experimentation abilities: learners 'must be able to use these theories to make decisions and solve problems'.[5] (p. 30)

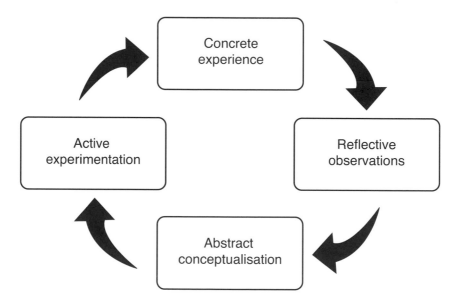

FIGURE 1.5 Kolb's Experiential Learning Cycle

For an example of the process of experiential learning I will turn to my two-year-old daughter who, as mentioned, discovered that goats 'baa' in a similar manner to sheep. I know this is hardly adult learning but it is a neat, simple example of experiential learning in action. So, on our trip to the farm, I can certainly vouch for her engagement with the experience and feel that she participated fully in the day's activities. One of the best things about parenthood is the reinvention of the mundane world around us. Perhaps to successfully achieve this first stage of the learning cycle we have to find our inner two-year-old, and approach life without the constraints of adult cynicism and fear of failure. The next stage of the learning cycle is reflective observation; can a two-year-old reflectively observe? Perhaps that's a discussion for another day, but at yesterday's bedtime and this morning she was chattering away about 'goat farm baa', 'sheep baa', 'stroke goat', 'goat baa' (anyone with children will recognise the circular nature of these conversations). So is she reflecting on the experience? I think as much as she is capable; she can't yet consider other perspectives (after all, what did the goat think about meeting her?), that particular skill will develop with age. Later this morning we got out her farm set to play with, and she picked up the sheep and the goat: 'baa'. The next step is abstract conceptualisation: she has taken the real life experience and is now applying it to the model that she is playing with. While she was playing, with a little help, she built a pen. Into that pen she put the sheep and the goat; they belong together because they make the same noise. She was experimenting with the new concept, putting it into the context of her world. Perhaps next time we go to a farm she will expect to find the goats in a pen with the sheep as she problem solves based on the new experience. Of course, if the goats are nowhere near the sheep, she will have to re-evaluate her initial hypothesis and find another way of classifying her farm animals.

There are some conflicts within the Experiential Learning Cycle (*see* Figure 1.6) because, in order to complete the cycle, the individual must possess skills that are contradictory in nature. The learner must expose themselves to concrete experiences but also conceptualise things in abstract contexts. They have to be reflective observers as well as being decision makers and problem solvers.

> Learning requires abilities that are polar opposites and the learner, as a result, must continually choose which set of learning abilities he or she will bring to bear in any specific learning situation.[5] (p. 34)

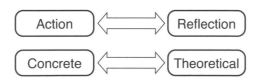

FIGURE 1.6 Learning skills conflicts in Kolb's Experiential Learning Cycle

The contradictory nature of the skills needed to complete the learning process adds to the challenge for the educator as well as the learner. We are asking the learner to master these very different skills and to recognise when to use them. Not an easy task and made almost impossible if we do not lend a helping hand in their development. However, in the context of Kolb's Experiential Learning Cycle, it is tricky to see exactly what the skills are. How do we help learners develop their ability to take on new concrete experiences? Or to abstractly conceptualise? There is some help to be found by looking at the work done by George Kelly.

Scientific inquiry and experiential learning

Kelly's[7] work is grounded in constructivism – linking experience and internal processes. He identified a similarity between the learning process and the process of scientific inquiry. His work was based upon the premise that people's psychological processes are scientific in nature and it has been incorporated into the Cognitive Behavioural Therapy movement. Kelly proposed the idea that every individual has a number of 'constructs' that are developed through personal experience. The very individualistic nature of these constructs means they can sometimes be a warped version of reality, but the differences are as a result of the individual's experiences. To take a very (very) simplistic example, someone who has been to the dentist once and had a horrible time has a 100% experience of a horrible time at the dentist. In truth, though, I know some very nice dentists. These constructs are used by the individual

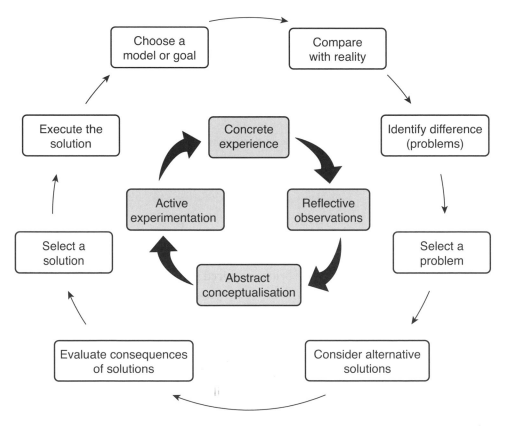

FIGURE 1.7 Kolb's Experiential Learning Cycle compared to the scientific process (as illustrated by Kolb)

to make predictions about likely outcomes of a particular behaviour. These hypotheses are then put to the test, through a combination of investing in and encountering the event. The actual outcome will either confirm or refute the initial hypothesis, which may require a revision of the original construct. So when the second trip to the dentist is not so bad after all, the initial hypothesis has been disproved and the individual has to review their future predictions. Essentially, this suggests that we can view thought processes as a series of mini scientific inquiries, often called the 'man as scientist' approach. It links closely with Piaget's[8] ideas of assimilation (the digestion of external factors to fit with internal constructs) and accommodation (the creation and adapting of internal constructs as a result of external factors). He links these ideas to another scientific process: that of equilibrium. Piaget describes our cognitive processes as equilibration – a process of constant exertions towards a cognitive equilibrium that will never be reached because there will always be new variables and influences.

To pull this into the experiential learning arena, we need a comparison of the scientific process with the Experiential Learning Cycle. Fortunately for us, Kolb did this as part of the development of his cycle (*see* Figure 1.7); he aligned the scientific process against the stages of his Experiential Learning Cycle.

Using the process of scientific inquiry as a lens to view experiential learning materialises the necessary skills in a more tangible form so we can see more clearly what we must help our learners to develop if they are to become self-directed.

Limitations of the Skills Pillar

It first has to be noted that, like much of adult education literature, research into experiential learning is almost entirely based in Western culture. This cultural bias in the research may or may not be of significance to the construction of the Skills Pillar, but it must certainly be taken into consideration. This three pillar model has been developed to help educators work with the learner(s) that are in front of them; at each step I would ask that educators consider their learners as unique individuals. The skills bricks that are uncovered throughout the rest of this book will not all be applicable to all learners, as the bricks required will depend on their personality, current skills, previous experiences and the learning context. Keeping this in mind should help to minimise the cultural bias issue that arises when attempting to draw conclusions for broader, mixed groups of learners.

As has already been briefly mentioned, the separate and sequential nature of the stages of Kolb's cycle is perhaps unrealistic for a work-based learning environment. However, for our Skills Pillar it is the skills needed for experiential learning that matter not the order in which they are used. If, in reality, workplace learning does not happen in this nice sequential and step-wise manner it does not matter as long as the learners have all the necessary skills. If a learner can successfully predict, reflect, problem solve, evaluate and so on, they will be able to negotiate a more chaotic learning environment.

One of the key criticisms of Kolb's Experiential Learning Cycle is that reflection is a single step in the cycle. As we shall see in Chapter 5, reflection is more complex than this. For this model of self-directedness, Kolb's learning cycle is being used as the overarching structure for the pillar; it is not an end point but a beginning. There are many possible bricks to be added to build the reflection skills needed for this section of the Skills Pillar.

The Skills Pillar: summary

The Skills Pillar is primarily constructed around Kolb's Experiential Learning Cycle[5] (*see* Figure 1.8), and in the subsequent chapters of this book we will uncover the tools and strategies that adult educators can utilise to develop the learning skills of a self-directed learner. We will be looking for anything that may help us to achieve the following for our learners.

Learners who:

- are open to new experiences and able to overcome the natural risk averseness of many adult learners
- can approach new experiences and opportunities without prejudice or cynicism
- have the insight to recognise the most effective learning experiences for their learning preferences
- are able and willing to take control of their learning environment to maximise the effectiveness of their learning experience
- understand how their learning applies to their prospective workplace
- have deep insight into themselves as a learner and as a person
- can make genuine and unbiased observations of the situation
- reflect usefully on their observations using a combination of internal and external perspectives
- reflect at a high cognitive level, synthesising information, evaluating perspectives and justifying their values
- problem solve creatively to generate a range of solutions
- critically consider the potential implications of different approaches
- use theoretical models to contextualise their own learning and learning needs
- set targets with clear outcomes
- identify their own learning needs in response to new experience or new information
- are capable of managing, organising and executing their plans
- can produce specific and achievable action plans to meet identified learning needs
- can evaluate the success of changes to their practice.

This pillar represents the importance of providing the learner with the tools, strategies and techniques necessary to allow them to successfully negotiate the learning process in a self-directed manner. Learners need the skills to learn and an insight into their strengths and weaknesses with regards to the learning cycle. This must be combined with a motivation to learn and an insight into their motivations – therefore motivation will be the second pillar of self-directedness.

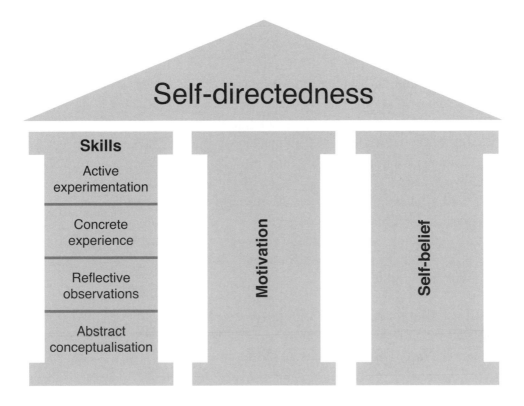

FIGURE 1.8 The Skills Pillar

THE MOTIVATION PILLAR

Thus far we have discussed the importance of providing learners with the necessary skills for self-directed learning. In the second pillar we will consider the motivation needed to encourage a learner to be self-directed. Motivation is an intensely personal thing, and we all have very different motivations that we may or may not be willing to share with others. However, the very individualistic nature of motivation does not prevent us from working to find the right 'buttons' and to develop a learner motivated towards lifelong learning.

There are many models of motivation and some of these will be discussed in greater detail in Chapter 7 when we look for the bricks that an educator can put in place to construct the Motivation Pillar. Given the nature of this model of self-directedness, we need a broad and all-encompassing model to provide the structure for this pillar, one that looks at all aspects of motivation, internal and external, personal and shared. We need a model that allows us to consider all aspects of the individual. We will, therefore, be using Maslow's Hierarchy of Needs[9] as the overall structure for the Motivation Pillar. Maslow's model encompasses a broad range of motivations that we can consider when putting in place mechanisms to motivate our learners in the immediate future and towards lifelong learning.

Maslow is seen as a humanistic psychologist; he viewed behaviours through the eyes of the individual, rather than through the eyes of an observer. Humanistic psychologists study behaviour as a consequence of the person as a whole. This is in contrast to the behaviourist approach that focuses on external triggers; the individual behaviour is as a result of the nature of the stimulus not their internal processes. However, Maslow did not ignore the behaviourist approach; indeed he incorporated ideas from behaviourism as well as humanism, biological theories, social theories, psychological theories (both child and adult) and anthropological theories to build his model. This individualistic yet holistic approach to motivation combines an understanding of the motivations that our learners may have in common with an understanding that the specific motivations may vary. Maslow's model will, therefore, provide structure around which educators can select the appropriate bricks for their individual learner.

Maslow's Hierarchy of Needs: the five-tier model

Maslow tentatively proposed his model for motivation in 1943,[9] when he published his untested theory for discussion and further research. As a model for motivation it has become widely accepted and published and can be found in most education, psychology and management textbooks.

Essentially the model is a five-tier pyramid (*see* Figure 1.9) constructed of the differing needs of an individual: physiological, safety, belongingness, self-esteem and self-actualisation. Maslow called the first four of these deficiency needs or D needs. These are things that we find ourselves in need of, that we will be motivated to find if we do not have them because we feel their absence as a deficiency in some way. The highest level of motivation is different because we do not notice the absence of self-actualisation. Instead this is a growth need, this is our capacity and our desire for growth, for personal improvement to become better in who we are and at what we do. We will now look more closely at each of the levels of Maslow's model to give us a greater understanding of the Motivation Pillar.

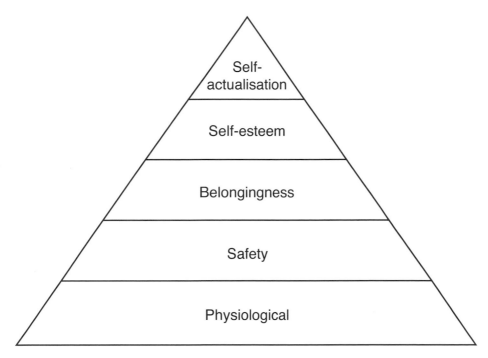

FIGURE 1.9 Maslow's Hierarchy of Needs

Physiological

At the bottom of the pyramid lies the most base of all needs, the physiological needs. Maslow used this level to identify the biological, often homeostatically controlled, aspects of motivation: the need for food (and indeed specific nutrition types), water, sex. There is a certain amount of controversy over the inclusion of 'sex' as a basic need. Depends on your perspective I suppose. These are the drives that motivate animals on the daily hunt for food and water. If these needs are not met, an individual will not go on to seek greater things as all their efforts, their thoughts and actions are guided by the need for food or water. It is by finding ways to secure our supply of these needs that we are able to move forward as a society.

Safety

If the physiological needs are met, an individual will find themselves driven by the need to be safe and secure. The marooned man on an island first finds food and water (maybe not sex) and will then move on to look for somewhere safe to sleep at night to avoid whatever sharp-toothed delights await him in the jungle. Maslow draws on research with children for this level as this is when it can be most clearly seen. The child who encounters an unknown or unusual situation, the child who is scared or poorly, will respond as if they are in danger and their response will be that of seeking safety. For most healthy, happy children, this safety is to be found with their protector, their parents, and the child will become clingy until they feel they are safe. This does not mean that safety-related motivations are irrelevant to adults, as there are many similar things that can provoke a safety need in adults; public speaking, for example, will leave many adults quivering in a corner asking for Mummy. It is also important to note that, for many people, children and adults, security can be found in routines, in the known and expected. For educators this is perhaps the most significant aspect of this level.

Belonging

The third of the deficiency needs is the need to be loved and be able to love. The sense of belonging is important in terms of personal relationships but also in terms of belonging to larger groups and communities. Once an individual has had their physiological and safety needs fulfilled, they can begin to focus on the need for loving relationships. The well-fed and well-protected man will look for relationships that are personal and intimate as well as wider relationships; he will want to feel part of a network, part of a community. The need for affectionate relationships will be a key motivator for some people; however, in the education context it may not be appropriate for this relationship to arise between educator and learner. Do not discount this motivational level, though, as there are other ways within our influence that we can ensure our learners feel part of a community.

Self-esteem

The highest of the deficiency needs proposed by Maslow is self-esteem. By labelling this as a deficiency need Maslow suggests we will be motivated by the absence of self-esteem. He divides this level of the hierarchy into two subsidiary levels:

> [Firstly,] the desire for strength, for achievement, for adequacy, for confidence in the face of the world, and for independence and freedom. Secondly, we have what we may call the desire for reputation or prestige (defining it as respect or esteem from other people), recognition, attention, importance or appreciation.[9] (pp. 382–3)

A high level of self-esteem leads to a feeling of self-worth. If these needs remain unmet the individual can feel (at best) mediocre and discouraged.

Self-actualisation

The peak of Maslow's hierarchy, self-actualisation, is the one and only growth need in this five-tier model. Once the deficiency needs have been met, individuals become motivated by a need to fulfil their potential. You may have seen this: that person who appears to have everything in terms of physiological and safety needs met, they have loving relationships and are held in high esteem by themselves and others, yet they are still restless for something more.

> A musician must make music, an artist must paint, a poet must write, if he is to be ultimately happy. What a man can be, he must be.[9] (p. 383)

The requirements for self-actualisation will vary widely from one person to another depending on how they view their life's purpose. It may be music, art, poetry or perhaps sporting or academic achievements or they may be motivated by being a good parent. Whatever the ultimate self-actualising need for the individual, this is a very powerful motivator and an important one to tap into if we are to develop self-directed learners.

Maslow's hierarchy of needs and today's society

Maslow proposed that an individual will be driven by the lowest unmet need. A desperately hungry person will be motivated by the search for food:

> The urge to write poetry, the desire to acquire an automobile, the interest in American history, the desire for a new pair of shoes are, in the extreme case, forgotten or become of secondary importance. For the man who is extremely and dangerously hungry, no other interests exist but food. He dreams food, he remembers food, he thinks about food, he emotes only about food, he perceives only food and he wants only food.[9] (pp. 374–5)

In our modern, Western society, desperate hunger of this nature is uncommon, and concerns around meeting physiological needs are more likely to be due to financial troubles. In the learning environment we will most likely find that our physiological needs are less extreme – related to temperature, light, room arrangements. We should also feel secure in our safety needs, for the main part, as long as we avoid dark alleys, we live in a relatively safe environment. There are no lions creeping up on us in our sleep. Maslow discussed the nature of safety needs in the modern society:

> The healthy, normal, fortunate adult in our culture is largely satisfied in his safety needs. The peaceful, smoothly running, 'good' society ordinarily makes its members feel safe enough from wild animals, extremes of temperature, criminals, assault and murder, tyranny, etc.[9] (pp. 379–80)

We need only Google 'dating sites' and consider the impact of social networking to see that the need for a sense of belonging is relevant in our society. Although the electronic age is changing relationships we certainly still need them and seek them in increasingly more complex ways.

The final deficiency need, self-esteem, resonates with many as being a fundamental need. The regular discussion of the impact of media on self-esteem of men, women and children is testament to the relevance in today's society. Increasing pressure to 'have it all' – friends, family and career – can easily lead to individuals feeling second rate for not achieving the hat-trick. With ever wider circles of comparison and social media streams filled with people showing how wonderful their life is, it can be easy to feel inferior.

Self-actualisation, being the only growth need in this version of the model, is very important for all educators. It is this need that we must tap into if we are to successfully motivate our learners to become self-directed. The hierarchical nature of Maslow's pyramid indicates that we must ensure the other, deficiency, needs are met before we can encourage our learners to truly and absolutely go in search of personal growth and become a self-actualising person.

Maslow's Hierarchy of Needs extended

The most well-known version of Maslow's Hierarchy of Needs is the original five-tier model he proposed in 1943.[9] However, when Maslow developed this original model he had not finished refining it. Over the following years he became increasing concerned that the top tier, self-actualisation, actually related to more than the 'self'. He began to see that self-actualisation may not be the only growth need to be found at the top of the hierarchy once the lower levels were met. There was something more because even those who were fulfilled, safe, loved and able to achieve their desired potential were still seeking more. These people are still motivated by some other, unidentified factor. So Maslow[10] took the idea of self-actualisation and went further to describe self-transcendence; he began to suggest a restructuring of the growth needs.

> I have recently found it more and more useful to differentiate between two kinds (or better, degrees) of self-actualizing people, those who were clearly healthy, but with little or no experience of transcendence, and those in whom transcendent experiencing was important and even central.[10 (p. 270)]

Maslow was indicating another level of growth needs, something else that should sit atop the four deficiency needs: self-transcendence (*see* Figure 1.10). He was unclear about how the two growth needs should be arranged, expressing some concerns regarding the hierarchical nature of these two needs. However, self-transcendence is usually represented as another level to be added to the top of the five tiers initially proposed, and it is one that is of great importance to the adult learning world.

Consider, why we are motivated to educate? Is it the pay and conditions? Hmmm, unlikely. The self-transcendence tier of Maslow's hierarchy suggests that some of us are motivated by a need to connect with others in a manner detached from the 'self'. This includes spiritual and religious connections as implied by the name. However, Maslow, himself an atheist, considered this level of self-transcendence to include more than religious altruism. It includes all altruistic acts, it incorporates collectivism into an otherwise individualistic model. There will be people who find themselves selflessly motivated to develop and maintain a unified connectedness with those around them. We can observe this type of self-transcendent behaviour in a parent with their child – more than a relationship that would be part of the 'belonging' level of the hierarchy, there is a need to give, both mentally and emotionally. An educational example would include those who offer to mentor colleagues with no incentive other than their own motivations. It represents a stage in a person's development where their sense of self comes second to a wider contribution.

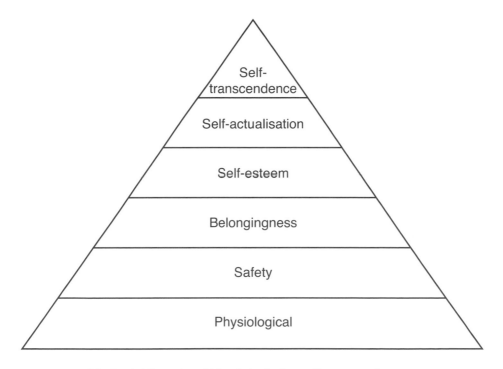

FIGURE 1.10 Maslow's Hierarchy of Needs including self-transcendence

Koltko-Rivera[11] discussed the loss of the self-transcendence tier from most publications of Maslow's Hierarchy of Needs and identified a number of reasons for its absence. He suggests a combination of unfortunate timing, poor communication and a lack of readiness for the concept in the psychology world. Whatever the reason for its continued absence from most textbooks, the self-transcendence level will be included in the structure of the Motivation Pillar as its importance in adult education should be recognised.

Limitations of the Motivation Pillar

Concerns have been raised regarding the cultural bias of Maslow's hierarchy. Hofstede[12] conducted research on the differences between individualistic and collectivistic cultures, including a consideration of Maslow's Hierarchy of Needs.

> The ordering of needs in Maslow's hierarchy represents a value choice – Maslow's value choice. This choice was based on his mid-twentieth century U.S. middle class values. First Maslow's hierarchy reflects individualistic values, putting self-actualisation and autonomy on top. Values prevalent in collective cultures, such as 'harmony' or 'family support,' do not even appear in the hierarchy. Second, the cultural map [developed by Hofstede] suggests even if just the needs Maslow used in his hierarchy are considered – the needs will have to be ordered differently in different cultural areas.[12 (p. 396)]

As previously stated in the discussion of the limitations of Kolb's Experiential Learning Cycle, this model is intended to be related to the individual learner. Only those aspects that are relevant to the unique learner should be applied; the decision about relevance lies with the skilled and thoughtful educator and cultural issues have to be part of their consideration.

Repeatedly, throughout the literature, different researchers identify concerns with the rigid hierarchical nature of the familiar pyramid (e.g. Wahba and Bridwell[13]). The model is often presented as a fixed and rigid hierarchy, but even in his initial introduction Maslow identified a number of exceptions where the levels were adapted for individuals: for example, those people where the need for self-esteem came before the need for love. Another, less common example is those people who are often held up as martyrs – they forgo all the most basic of needs for the sake of a particular value or ideal. As well as these variations for the lower growth needs, Maslow also had issues with the hierarchical nature of the top needs of self-actualisation and self-transcendence that he could not resolve before his death.

For our Three Pillar Model of Self-directedness we need to question the significance of that hierarchical nature of Maslow's model. The Hierarchy of Needs will provide a structure for the Motivation Pillar, within which we can organise the bricks we will find to build the pillar. The specific bricks required will vary depending on the individual and will be identified by skilled educators who know their learners. We can, therefore, take the hierarchical nature of the model with a pinch of salt. We can use it to identify different aspects of motivation and even to identify the main motivational needs at any one time for a specific learner. There does not need to be a hierarchy to see that a learner experiencing a messy divorce may have greater safety and security needs, or financial troubles may cause all motivations to revert to getting food on the table. There is a significant amount of research that supports the hierarchy so we need not fully discount it when looking at the structure of this pyramid. We should just approach it with caution and consider the individual in front of us before the pyramid, rather than the other way around.

The Motivation Pillar – a summary

The Motivation Pillar is organised according to Maslow's Hierarchy of Needs, including the highest level added later on: self-transcendence (*see* Figure 1.11). In the rest of this book we will uncover the things that educators can do to develop learner motivation and learner insight into their motivations. The former is important for self-directedness in the immediate future of their formalised learning, while the latter will be important for learners to continue to be self-directed after the formal learning process. We will be looking for strategies and structures that educators can employ to achieve the following outcomes.

Learners who:

- can ensure their physiological needs are met within their workplace or learning environment
- recognise their own insecurities and know how to deal with them
- can develop a feeling of safety and security in their workplace or learning environment
- are able to identify the need for help and ask for the relevant helpful information
- are able to exist as part of a community
- have the ability to build positive relationships with peers and colleagues
- develop positive relationships with mentors (formal or informal)
- are confident in themselves and who hold a high level of self-worth
- have a good reputation and who are held in high esteem by their colleagues
- are secure enough in themselves to seek out feedback and take criticism constructively
- are able to recognise personal achievement and accept encouragement and praise
- are able to fulfil their potential and meet their desired goals
- hold a strong belief in the value of a self-directed approach for the achievement of their personal goals
- understand how their working and learning preferences will impact their ability to be self-directed
- have the insight into their personal motivations to allow them to pursue their personal goals
- are able to move beyond the confines of their own lives to seek out information to illuminate and enrich their knowledge of their chosen goals

- have a metacognitive understanding of themselves
- see themselves as part of a wider context
- recognise and embrace the nature of an unknown future with unknown challenges.

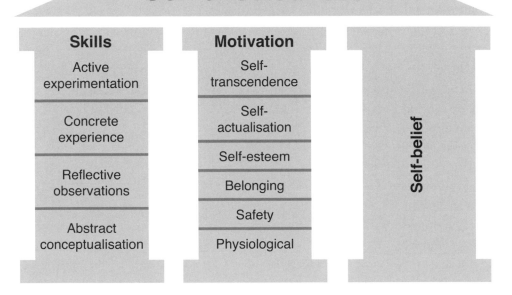

FIGURE 1.11 The Motivation Pillar

This pillar represents a very personal aspect of self-directedness: motivation. While the individualistic nature of the skills identified in the first pillar is important, for this pillar it is even more so. Every learner will be different in terms of which deficiency needs have been met and the requirements needed to meet them. The growth needs of self-actualisation and self-transcendence are also unique to the individual. So the educator must make skilled judgements of the bricks they need to include in this pillar for their specific learner, rather than try to include all the available bricks or make standardised responses.

THE SELF-BELIEF PILLAR

Once we have instilled in our learners the necessary skills for learning and the motivation to carry out the learning behaviour there is still one more aspect to consider that is often omitted. Our learner is willing and able to be self-directed in their learning, but they must believe they are capable of achieving it. This is their self-belief. Without it a learner is unlikely to attempt a particular task. The learner knows how to do it (whatever 'it' may be) and has sufficient motivations pushing or pulling them to do it, but they don't have the self-belief that they can do it so they talk themselves out of even attempting it. While self-belief and motivation are closely linked, there is a subtle but important distinction to be made. A learner may be very motivated but without the belief that they are capable of being successful the strength of the motivational factors becomes irrelevant.

Vroom's[14] expectancy theory is a motivation theory that suggests the impetus for action is a result of a combination of three things:

1. the expectancy that a performance will lead to the desired outcome
2. the expectancy that the individual's effort will lead to the required performance and
3. the valence – how highly the individual values the outcome.

Without the expectation that completing a particular course will be educative, enjoyable, a networking opportunity or good on their CV, the behaviour will seem pointless to the learner. However, it is the second of Vroom's factors that is very closely linked to self-efficacy – the belief that the individual is capable of effectively completing the behaviour. If the learner does not believe they can successfully complete the course, even if they know it will improve their CV, they will not go ahead and enrol (*see* Figure 1.12). It is self-efficacy, as described by Bandura,[15] that will provide the structure for our third pillar of self-directedness.

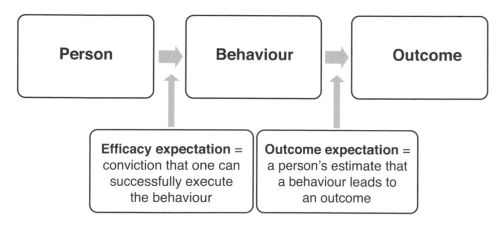

FIGURE 1.12 Efficacy and outcome expectations (as described by Bandura)

Bandura[15] has contributed perhaps the most well-recognised theory of self-efficacy: Social Cognitive Theory. Much of Bandura's work had roots in behaviourism (look it up – some rather unusual experiments involving women and children punching

Bobo dolls. Seriously). However, in developing his Social Cognitive Theory, he recognised that research was beginning to shift the emphasis towards a more individualistic (more humanistic) approach to behaviours.

> Reinterpretation of antecedent determinants as predicative cues, rather than as controlling stimuli, has shifted the locus of the regulation of behaviour from the stimulus to the individual.[15 (p. 192)]

That is, a single stimulus will produce different behaviours in different people, and the cause of the behaviour is not determined by the stimulus itself but by the way it is perceived by the individual. After all, we don't all run screaming from spiders.

In this theory Bandura recognised the importance of cognitive processes in determining how the individual perceives the stimulus. He saw that the immediate behavioural response to a stimulus may be further processed cognitively over a long period of time. Therefore, his seminal work (Social Cognitive Theory) was, as the name suggests, cognitively based. He also proposed that while the individual is shaped by their environment, the environment is also shaped by the individual in a process he called reciprocal determinism, which is part of the 'social' element of his Social Cognitive Theory.

We will use Bandura's Social Cognitive Theory as the structure for the final pillar: Self-belief. The individual, as a unique person, is placed right at the heart of this theory but with consideration of input from external factors. This combination of internal and external meshes nicely with Maslow's motivational theory and with the combination of externally sourced experiences and internal processing found in Kolb's learning cycle.

Self-efficacy

There are various 'self' terms out there that become increasingly difficult to separate from one another: self-belief, self-concept, self-worth, self-image, self-efficacy. There are subtle differences between them but also a number of similarities, especially if we ask the question 'How do we improve a person's self-belief/self-concept/self-worth/self-image/self-efficacy?' Since we are viewing these ideas from the perspective of the educational front line, we don't really need to get bogged down in a discussion of the minutiae of these definitions. Instead we will look just at one that is of particular interest to educators working to develop self-directed learners: self-efficacy. Self-efficacy is an individual's belief in how successfully they can complete a task. Therefore, in the context of this model, it is reasonable to use self-efficacy as a substitute for self-belief. We are considering the individual's level of self-belief in a learning context, and this requires learners to believe they can successfully complete the learning goals they have set for themselves.

An individual with a high level of self-efficacy is both more likely to attempt the task and more likely to continue to persist when obstacles arise. This latter point is particularly important as an individual who persists and achieves will raise their level of self-efficacy while those who give up will reinforce their low self-efficacy.

> The stronger the perceived self-efficacy, the more active the efforts. Those who persist in subjectively threatening activities that are in fact relatively safe will gain corrective experiences that reinforce their sense of efficacy, thereby eventually eliminating their defensive behaviour. Those who cease their coping efforts prematurely will retain their self-debilitating expectations and fear for a long time.[15 (p. 194)]

Attribution theory provides more detail on the implication of failure, and the individual's perception of the reason for the failure will be important. An external locus for the failure will have less of an impact than if the individual believes they were responsible or lacking in some way.

Bandura was careful to qualify his theory with the recognition that a high level of self-efficacy is not the sole determinant of behaviour. However, it is certainly a major contributor. Sabagghian[16] reached a similar conclusion linking self-image and self-directedness.

> There is a strong relationship between the self-image of adult students and their self-directedness in learning. As adults gain the ability to direct and organise their own learning they consider themselves more and more as worthy persons in every aspect of life. Adult students with higher self-concepts appear to be … more likely to be able to plan and direct the majority of their learning projects themselves than adult students with lower self-concepts.[16 (pp. 114–15)]

We have so far introduced self-efficacy as if it were a single entity when in fact it is nowhere near as simple (nothing ever is). There are actually three dimensions in which a person's self-efficacy may vary: magnitude, generality and strength. A large magnitude of self-efficacy will allow the learner to take on even the most difficult tasks, whereas smaller magnitudes of self-efficacy would limit the individual to attempting only simple tasks. There will be some experiences that create a very general self-efficacy, a belief in their abilities that allows them to attempt tasks that are novel and different to those previously undertaken. However, some experiences will be much more specific to the type of task. Finally, levels of self-efficacy may vary in their strength. In some areas an individual may have a strong level of self-efficacy, which will allow them to continue in the face of adversity and which will be more robust in the face of failure. However, other areas may be weak so the individual will quickly give up and will find their self-efficacy in this area easily undermined. All this leads us to a rather complex model of self-efficacy. Fortunately for us Bandura laid out four sources of self-efficacy that we can use to structure our thoughts about how to increase the magnitude, generality and strength of our learner's self-efficacy.

Social Cognitive Theory

Self-efficacy theories vary in their descriptions of how levels of efficacy are determined. In social learning theory people learn from others and their level of self-efficacy is based upon their belief that they can contribute to a group setting. In self-concept theory self-efficacy is based upon successes and failures and other information received from external sources. Attribution theory looks at how people react differently to causes attributed internally or externally. In this theory an internal locus for the cause of the event will lead to greater levels of self-efficacy, whereas an external locus for a failed event may lead to feelings of humiliation and anger.

There are four mechanisms through which self-efficacy levels may be raised or lowered:

- performance accomplishments
- vicarious experience
- verbal persuasion
- emotional arousal.

The first and most effective source of efficacy is 'performance accomplishments'. Unsurprisingly, successful performances will raise an individual's self-efficacy level while failures will lower it. Most educators cannot class themselves as psychologists, but I think it is fair to say all have some interest in 'the person' in the learning context. As such most would have reached this conclusion as a result of their own experiences. Where Bandura's research goes further is in the details of the link between self-efficacy levels and performance accomplishments.

> After strong efficacy expectations are developed through repeated success, the negative impact of occasional failures is likely to be reduced. Indeed occasional failures that are later overcome by determined effort can strengthen self-motivated persistence if one finds through experience that even the most difficult obstacles can be mastered by sustained effort. ... Once established, enhanced self-efficacy tends to generalise to other situations. ... However, the generalisation effects occur most predictably to the activities that are most similar.[15] (pp. 195–6)

Bandura identified a number of modes of induction for performance accomplishments; these are the ways in which we can use 'performance accomplishments' to raise self-efficacy.

- Participant modelling – provide opportunities for the learner to carry out the successful actions in a modelled scenario with guidance from the educator.
- Performance desensitisation – expose the learner repeatedly to anxiety-inducing events, gradually increasing the level of perceived difficulty of the exposure. This would usually be combined with relaxation techniques at each stage.
- Performance exposure – provide opportunities for the learner to be exposed to the perceived risky situations in a prolonged and highly anxiety-inducing manner until the individual no longer exhibits anxiety in the situation.
- Self-instructed performance – encourage the learner to instigate events. Successful self-directedness will breed more self-directedness.

The second source of self-efficacy is 'vicarious experience' – we gain self-belief by seeing others, particularly peers similar to ourselves, achieve successes. This is a less powerful source of self-efficacy for the learner because the information gained does not directly relate to their own personal capabilities. There are a number of considerations for this source of self-efficacy. First, it has been shown that people benefit more from seeing others achieve through persistent effort than from seeing proficient individuals succeed at a task with ease. Second, the effect of this source can be increased by providing the opportunity for the learner to observe achievement by a diverse selection of people. The learner begins to believe that if all those different people can do it, so can they. Third, the learner needs to see clear outcomes from their observations of other people's behaviours.

Bandura also identified modes of induction for this source of efficacy.

- Live modelling – provide opportunities for the learner to observe someone else modelling the successful behaviours.
- Symbolic modelling – provide opportunities for the learner to observe videos, photographs and the like of others achieving success.

The third source of self-efficacy is 'verbal persuasion', which is less powerful than both performance accomplishments and vicarious experience. This is a relatively weak source of efficacy because it does not actually demonstrate success; self-belief built upon verbal persuasion is easily extinguished. As educators, the previous two sources of self-efficacy are about providing carefully designed opportunities with appropriate guidance. This third source relates more to the behaviour of the educator themselves. The key to effective use of this source of efficacy is to use it in combination with the skills necessary to complete the task successfully, in this case the learning skills identified for the Skills Pillar.

> People who are socially persuaded that they possess the capabilities to master difficult situations and are provided with provisional aids for effective action are likely to

> mobilise greater effort than those who receive only the performance aids. However, to raise by persuasion expectations of personal competence without arranging conditions to facilitate effective performance will most likely lead to failures that discredit the persuaders and further undermine the recipients' perceived self-efficacy.[15 (p. 198)]

Raising expectations through verbal persuasion without putting the necessary skills structure for success in place will not only result in efficacy-reducing failures but can also undermine the persuader in the eyes of the individual.

There are four modes of induction for verbal persuasion suggested by Bandura.

- Suggestion – the educator should indicate and signpost a suitable goal.
- Exhortation – the educator should also give stronger encouragement, urging the learner into action towards a goal.
- Self-instruction – the educator should facilitate situations in which the learner's internal monologue persuades them into action.
- Interpretive treatments – provide opportunities that are revealing for the learner and allow them to develop the internal monologue necessary for self-instruction.

Finally, the weakest source of self-efficacy is 'emotional arousal'. You may have experienced this situation yourselves, when you get so worked up and anxious about a particular event you exhibit physiological signs of stress. It is likely that this heightened state of arousal will impair your performance, so the ability to relax under these conditions is more likely to lead to success.

> By conjuring up fear-provoking thoughts about their ineptitude, individuals can rouse themselves to elevated levels of anxiety that far exceed the fear experiences during the actual threatening situation.[15 (p. 199)]

It should be noted that sometimes, to some degree and for some people, this increased emotional arousal can actually result in better performance. Therefore, at the risk of repeating myself, it is important to strike the correct balance for the individual in front of you rather than applying a broad brushstroke.

Even though this is a very weak source of self-efficacy it still has an important role in adult education. For example, it could be particularly important if there are exam performances or public presentations to be considered. As Bandura states, 'diminishing emotional arousal can reduce avoidance behaviour';[15 (p. 199)] therefore it is important for self-directedness that we work to remove this potential barrier for our learners to approach new experiences openly. There are four modes of induction to increase self-efficacy through reducing emotional arousal.

- Attribution – there are two possible mechanisms to use attribution, though both are weak:

  ○ encourage the learner to believe that the anxiety-inducing event cannot affect them internally
  ○ provide misdirection so that the learner comes to attribute the anxiety to an alternative source.
- Relaxation, biofeedback – help the learner to reduce their anxieties of perceived risky behaviour through physical relaxation techniques.
- Symbolic desensitisation – provide opportunities to gradually increase exposure to the feared situation through symbolic means such as videos or photographs.
- Symbolic exposure – provide opportunities for sustained, maximum exposure to the perceived risky behaviours through videos or photographs.

Limitations of the Self-belief Pillar

First, it should be reiterated that we are using the mechanisms suggested by Bandura to raise self-efficacy (the belief that the learner can succeed) to structure what we are calling the 'self-belief' pillar. However, as we are essentially trying to answer the question 'How can we raise self-belief to improve self-directedness?' the comparison is reasonable. In our context, the meaning of 'self-belief' is what Bandura defines as 'self-efficacy'.

Second, while this model is looking at the individual's self-efficacy or self-belief and therefore the individual's self-directedness, it is important to note that there is a thing known as 'collective efficacy'. A person working as part of a group may buy into a sense of group self-belief – a belief that they, as a group, are capable (or not) of achieving a task. The achievements or failures of the group will likely impact upon the individual's level of self-efficacy if they feel their input has contributed to the success or failure. In fact, Singh[17] identified an increase in self-directedness of individuals after they were part of group achievements in the workplace. However, the sense of efficacy they demonstrate as part of the group may not reflect their true individual level of self-belief.

Finally, Bandura himself points out that a high level of self-efficacy is not a sole determinant of attempting a task. In this model, self-belief is just one of three pillars that are required to encourage self-directedness in learning, so we are not considering self-efficacy in isolation from other aspects.

The Self-belief Pillar: a summary

In order to complete our model of self-directedness we have put in place the third and final pillar. The Self-belief Pillar is based upon Bandura's Social Cognitive Theory[15] that identifies four sources of information for educators and learners in building up the learners' level of self-efficacy (*see* Figure 1.13). It is equally as important as the first two pillars; without a high level of self-belief it is unlikely a learner will become self-directed. Instead they will need constant nudging and pushing by their educators to complete the requirements for their current learning, and may deliberately shun future learning opportunities. To avoid this dependent behaviour we will hunt through relevant literature to identify the bricks we can put in place to build up the learner's level of self-efficacy according to the structure laid out by Bandura. We will undertake a systematic search to achieve the following outcomes for our learners.

Learners who:

- are able to set themselves appropriate goals that are both challenging and achievable
- can use past successes as a stimulus for future actions
- have the tools to negotiate and structure the external and internal information available to them to ensure success
- can use feedback to build success
- are able to identify successful learning processes in others and have the insight to apply these to themselves
- actively seek out valuable opportunities for observing others
- are aware of the nature of the supportive relationships they build

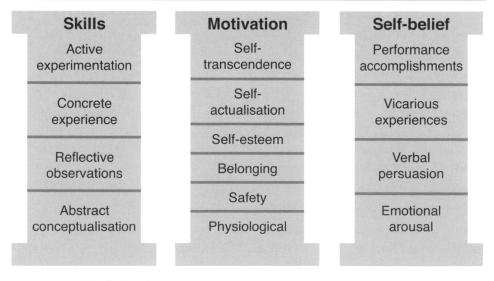

FIGURE 1.13 The Self-belief Pillar

- have the insight to recognise traits in their mentors that are key to their impact on the development of the learner
- have the insight into their emotional state and the impact it has on their ability to succeed
- are equipped to manage their level of emotional arousal in anxiety-inducing situations
- can, when appropriate, tackle anxiety-inducing challenges head on
- can build their confidence by gradually exposing themselves to perceived risky situations.

USING THE THREE PILLAR MODEL OF SELF-DIRECTEDNESS

This model can be considered to have three layers of increasing complexity. The first is the overall, basic construction of three pillars: Skills, Motivation and Self-belief, holding up the learner's self-directedness. This is a simple, easy way of looking at the educational aspects that need to be in place to achieve self-directedness for our learners.

The second layer is the structure of each pillar (*see* Table 1.1). The Skills Pillar is made up of the four steps in Kolb's Experiential Learning Cycle[5] (concrete experience, reflective observation, abstract conceptualisation and active experimentation). The Motivation Pillar is constructed from the six levels of Maslow's Hierarchy of Needs[9] (physiological, safety, belongingness, self-esteem, self-actualisation and self-transcendence). The Self-belief Pillar is built around the four sources of self-efficacy from Bandura's Social Cognitive Theory[15] (performance accomplishments, vicarious experiences, verbal persuasion and emotional arousal). These models provide each pillar with a structure that allows us to organise our thoughts regarding each aspect of self-directedness.

The third and final layer to this model is the individual bricks that we, as educators, can put in place to build each of the pillars. These bricks will be the actual things that we can do to help our learners develop the skills, motivation and self-belief to become self-directed. The skills bricks describe what an educator can do to develop skills and learner insight to allow the learner to navigate Kolb's Experiential Learning Cycle. The motivation bricks describe what an educator can put in place to ensure their learner is motivated, now and in the future, at each level of Maslow's Hierarchy of Needs. The self-belief bricks describe how an educator can cultivate their learners' level of self-efficacy using the four sources described by Bandura in his Social Cognitive Theory. The bricks will be sourced from across educational, psychological and management literature and you will find you do not need to achieve all the bricks for every learner. The third layer of this diagram will be different for each learner as the educator uses their own knowledge and skills to identify the requirements for the unique individual they are working with. If we, as educators, can build up the bricks appropriate to our learners to construct each of these three pillars we can support our learners to become self-directed both in their current learning environment and as they move on to the rest of their career.

TABLE 1.1 The structure of the three pillars for self-directedness

Pillar	Theory	Categories
Skills Pillar	Kolb	Concrete experience
		Reflective observation
		Abstract conceptualisation
		Active experimentation
Motivation Pillar	Maslow	Physiological
		Safety
		Belongingness
		Self-esteem
		Self-actualisation
		Self-transcendence
Self-belief Pillar	Bandura	Performance accomplishments
		Vicarious experience
		Verbal persuasion
		Emotional arousal

USING THE BRICKS

Each brick is located in two places. First, it is in our model for developing self-directedness. Each brick will belong in one of the three pillars: Skills, Motivation, Self-belief. Within the pillar they will fit into one of the categories that have been determined by Kolb's,[5] Maslow's[9] and Bandura's[15] models respectively. They will be assigned a code depending on this location:

Skill bricks:

- Concrete experience (CE)
- Reflective observation (RO)
- Abstract conceptualisation (AC)
- Active experimentation (AE)

Motivation bricks:

- Self-transcendence (ST)
- Self-actualisation (SA)
- Self-esteem (SE)

- Belonging (B)
- Safety (S)
- Physiological (P)

Self-belief bricks:
- Performance accomplishments (PA)
- Vicarious experience (VE)
- Verbal persuasion (VP)
- Emotional arousal (EA)

Second, the bricks can be located according to the area of research from which they have been found:
- Self-directedness and Adult learning (SD)
- People and Places (PP)
- Mentoring and Coaching (MC)
- Learning and Teaching (LT)
- Reflective practice and Action research (RA)
- Leadership and Management (LM)

Each brick will also be given a number to locate further information within the relevant chapter. This is simply to allow us to easily find further detail about how the brick may help us develop self-directedness.

So, an example code would be Skills: **RO3**: RA5 (*see* Figure 1.14). This tells us that this is the third brick that relates to the development of reflective observation skills and that further information can be found in the Reflective practice and Action research chapter; this is the fifth brick in that chapter.

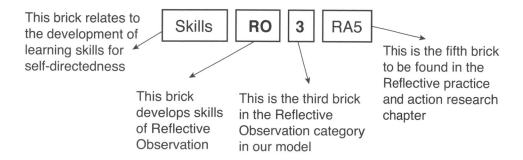

FIGURE 1.14 Coding the bricks

One of the keys to using this model successfully is to realise that the constituent parts of the pillars will vary depending on the educational context and the learner.

It is always important to consider the knowledge and skills of an individual since strengths and weaknesses will obviously vary from one person to another. Different people are motivated in different ways and may be strongly internally motivated or may require external factors to motivate them, but the need for an individual to have insight into their own motivations remains a constant. The level of self-efficacy that an individual has will be very individual and task related; it will depend on the types of past successes they have enjoyed or failures they have endured or overcome. Each of these variables will affect the way that a learner filters the words and actions of their educator and the way they perceive the impacts and outcomes of learning encounters. It comes down to the skill of the educator to identify what is most important for the unique combination of person and context in front of them.

The rest of this book is divided into sections of literature that will provide us with useful bricks for our pillars. We will cover the following areas that are derived from different sources of research:

- **Chapter 2: Self-directedness and adult learning:** the first, and most obvious, chapter looks at what we can learn from research into self-directedness so far and what adult learning has to teach us with regards to defining and developing self-directedness.

- **Chapter 3: People and places:** a closer look at the nature of the individual and the learning environment provided. This chapter will look for the bricks that can be put in place to develop the individual as well as provide the appropriate learning setting.

- **Chapter 4: Mentoring and coaching:** adult education often involves a mentor/ mentee or coach/coachee style of relationship. This chapter looks at how skills utilised in these similar yet opposing types of relationship can be used to develop self-directedness.

- **Chapter 5: Reflective practice and action research:** this chapter looks at reflection cycles and action research cycles to identify the skills and opportunities that can be used by adult educators to develop self-directedness.

- **Chapter 6: Learning and teaching:** this is another key aspect in any educational setting. This chapter will consider the teaching tools and techniques that are relevant to the adult learning context and the development of self-directedness.

- **Chapter 7: Leadership and management:** this is perhaps not an immediately obvious source for information but we are leading and managing the learning taking place and we want our learners to take over the leadership and management of their learning. There are, therefore, a number of useful theories and models to consider from this branch of research in looking for bricks to build our pillars.

CHAPTER 2

Self-directedness and adult learning

'Just as dependency and helplessness can be learned, self-direction can be learned – and it can be taught.'[1] (p. 127)

Gerald Grow

We begin our search for bricks by looking at the literature in the adult learning arena with specific reference to self-directedness: it would be inappropriate to begin anywhere else. There is already plenty of literature regarding self-directed learning; some is pretty abstract and some practical and easily applicable. Merriam[2] identified three strands to research into self-directedness: research into the goals of self-directed learning, research into the self-directed learner themselves, and research into the process of 'teaching' self-directed learning. Each of these areas of research will feed into our discussion to help us narrow down a definition of self-directedness. We will consider different aspects of the learner and their context to identify those factors that may impact upon the development of self-directedness. There are models regarding the teaching of self-directedness, and we will take a look at a couple of them to see how they can be built into our own instructional model for developing self-directedness.

A sensible starting point seems to be to define what we actually mean by self-directed learning. Our learners may all be different (in some cases wildly different), but surely it will be relatively easy to agree on what we want from a self-directed learner?

TOWARDS A DEFINITION OF SELF-DIRECTED LEARNING

The fundamental question is: What do we mean by self-directedness? In my experience learning conversations between adult educators on self-directed learning often revolve around questions like:

- Are all adult learners truly self-directed? Is self-directed learning synonymous with high achieving?
- Is self-directed learning a person-orientated personality trait? Or is it task orientated and dependent on the individual's personal interest and motivations in that area?
- If someone requires external motivators to begin tasks (e.g. 'It'll look good on your CV'), but is then completely independent in their learning, are they self-directed?
- How much do we expect from self-directed learners? Is self-directedness an all or nothing characteristic? Where on the spectrum between entirely independent and totally dependent do our expectations lie?
- How much do we adapt our vision of a self-directed learner based upon the individual in front of us? Are there cultural issues to be considered?

All of these are good questions and the discussions that take place in determining the answers are valuable and useful for the educators involved. You will find some answers within this book; for others it will provide background and information to add to the discussions as you reach your own personal conclusions.

There is one key conflict in defining self-directed learning: the context of the learning. Are we trying to define self-directedness in the formal classroom? The even more formal lecture theatre? Tutorials? The workplace? Single learning episodes? Long-term performance reviews? Therefore, before looking more closely at some definitions of self-directed learning we will briefly consider the context of the definitions. There are a considerable number of models that attempt to identify strands and dimensions to self-directed learning. Candy[3] divided current definitions of self-directedness into four dimensions:

- personal autonomy (self-direction as a personal quality)
- self-management (the individual's willingness and capacity to direct their learning)
- learner control (self-direction within a formal learning environment)
- autodidaxy (the more experiential, reflective practices of learning outside formal instruction).

Garrison[4] suggested that self-directed learning was the result of three interacting domains: self-management, self-monitoring and motivation.

Brockett and Hiemstra[5] collected the differing perspectives of self-directed learning into two areas. The first area is process; the learner takes control over planning and implementing in a formal setting. The second area is learner self-direction. This is a personality trait: the learner's desire to take responsibility for learning. They went on to suggest a model to encompass these differing views: The Personal Responsibility Orientation model, which we will look at a little later.

There are, therefore, two key qualities that we can aspire to develop in our learners. First, to develop learners who will take responsibility for their learning within our formalised learning context. Hand in hand with this, we are trying to develop learners who continue to learn after they have finished the course or graduated. Ideally, medical educators everywhere would be developing self-directedness in their learners and the NHS would be inundated with learners who can demonstrate personal autonomy, self-management, autodidaxy and learner control. They would seek out experiential learning opportunities, reflect upon and monitor their own performances, take control of their learning within formal settings and boldly go where no learner has gone before. Okay, so this perhaps borders on overly idealistic, but 'idealism' does not mean we should not aspire towards it; we have to accept that we cannot achieve all these skills for all learners but self-directedness is still a valuable and valued target.

Thus far we have discussed the different contexts in which to apply a definition, but we have not yet identified a specific description of self-directed learning. To achieve this, we need to look closer at the beginnings of andragogy (adult learning theory) and consider the ideas described by Knowles, who has earned himself the title of the 'father of andragogy'.

When Knowles[6] wrote *The Adult Learner: a neglected species* he used the term 'andragogy' (a word obtained from Yugoslavia apparently; there's something I didn't know) to describe the teaching of adult learners. His premise was that adult education was being damaged by adult educators attempting to teach adults using pedagogical ideas. Though this strict division of child versus adult teaching is now not considered as clear cut, he did propose a number of interesting assumptions for adult learning.

1. Changes in self-concept: 'As a person grows and matures his self-concept moves from one of total dependency (as is the reality of the infant) to one of increasing self-directedness.'[6] (p. 45)

2. The role of experience: In andragogy 'there is a decreasing emphasis on the transmittal techniques of traditional teaching and increasing emphasis on experiential techniques which tap the experience of the learners and involve them in analysing their experience.'[6] (p. 46) The importance of experiential learning has already been evidenced in our model by utilising Kolb's Experiential Learning Cycle as the structure for our Skills Pillar.

3. Readiness to learn: 'Andragogy assumes that learners are ready to learn those things they "need" to because of the developmental phases that are approaching

in the roles as workers, spouses, parents, organisational members and leaders, leisure time users and the like.'[6] (p. 47)

4. Orientation to learning: 'Adults tend to have a problem-centred orientation to learning as opposed to a subject-centred orientation.'[6] (p. 47)

While each of these has relevance to us as adult educators, the most interesting in terms of defining self-directedness is the development of self-concept. Knowles indicates that the need to be self-directed develops once an individual reaches 18 years old, though (as we shall discuss later) this is not so easily defined. Knowles recognises that some people feel a strong urge to take control of their learning while others feel much less inclined to manage their own development. However, he argues that the trait is always present in all adults, just not to the same degree. This assumption has been criticised because it is linear in its description of the development of self-directedness; it does not account for different settings and timings of a person's life. An individual returning to education after a period of time away from studying or work may be less inclined to be self-directed, at least initially, despite being older. Additionally, an individual may be very self-directed in one area of their lives but not in another. Perhaps what we can take from discussion of Knowles' adult learning theory is that self-direction is an inherent adult characteristic and it will be there (somewhere) in adult learners. However, we should not take it for granted especially if working with young adults. Knowles further develops his discussion of self-directedness in a later book: *Self-directed Learning: a guide for learners and teachers*.[7] In this text Knowles provides a clear and much repeated definition of self-directedness:

> A process in which individuals take the initiative, with or without the help of others, in diagnosing their learning needs, formulating goals, identifying human and other material resources for learning, choosing and implementing appropriate learning strategies, and evaluating learning outcomes.[7] (p. 18)

Brookfield[8] (another influential individual in adult education and particularly self-directed learning) has a slightly simpler but very similar definition.

> The process by which adults take control of their own learning, in particular how they set their own learning goals, locate appropriate resources, decide on which learning methods to use and evaluate their progress.[8]

The Knowles definition was expanded somewhat in 1991 by Hammond and Collins.[9]

> A process in which learners take the initiative, with the support and collaboration of others, for increasing self- and social-awareness; critically analysing and

reflecting on their situations; diagnosing their learning needs with specific reference to competencies they have helped identify; formulating socially and personally relevant learning goals; choosing and implementing appropriate learning strategies; and reflecting on and evaluating their learning. The immediate goal of critical self-directed learning is to help learners take control of their learning. Its ultimate goal is to empower learners to use their learning to improve the conditions under which they and those around them live and work.[9] (pp. 13–14)

In a review of self-directed learning models, Merriam and Caffarella[2] found that this definition by Hammond and Collins was the only one to include a broader social context to the concept. Other definitions, as seen here, focus on the individual's achievements.

It would be possible to trawl through the research and develop a long list of definitions. This would be without doubt one of the most mind-numbingly, brain-meltingly boring things you have ever read. It would also be unlikely to reward us with a consensus view of the detailed definition for self-directedness. The following definition is a combination of different ideas from the definitions already discussed. It is all-encompassing and just differs slightly from the previous discussion because it describes the learner rather than the process of self-directed learning. Since we are aiming to develop self-directedness as a trait in our learners it is appropriate to consider it from this slightly different angle.

> A self-directed learner will be able and willing to seek out learning opportunities and will hold the necessary belief in their own abilities to take control of their learning in formal and informal settings. They will identify suitable learning objectives given internal and external factors and work towards them in an effective manner using appropriate resources and strategies. They will then analyse, evaluate and reflect upon the outcomes of their learning in order to inform future learning opportunities.

Hopefully we are now clear on what we are aiming for, so now we need to start at the beginning and consider the readiness of the learner. Our learners are complex and complicated but somehow, with our guidance, they will hopefully find their way through their learning to meet their chosen objectives. Our challenge is to make sure they not only meet the required objectives but that they also develop the right combination of skills, motivation and self-belief to be self-directed in their approach to learning throughout their career. Easy!?

READINESS FOR SDL

Lesson one for educational change according Cox[10] is 'Readiness is a prior condition for change'[10 (p. 347)] and it seems perfectly rational to consider the readiness of our learners for self-directed learning. It should never be assumed that learners are ready for self-directed learning, and it would be a mistake to jump straight into a self-directed learning programme.

Age vs maturity

As has already been suggested from a discussion of Knowles' theory, and probably from anecdotal discussions among most adult educators, there are degrees of 'readiness' for self-directed learning. This is a significant area of research and the majority agreement seems to be that self-directedness is an aspect of personality that develops as a person matures.

> As an individual matures, his need and capacity to be self-directing, to utilise his experience in learning to identify his own readiness to learn, and to organise his learning around life problems, increases steadily from infancy to pre-adolescence and then, increasingly rapidly during adolescence'[6 (p. 43)]

Vygotsky[11] describes maturity as a change in the form of behaviour or as a shift from quantity to quality. Developmental research commonly defines specific age ranges for development of particular cognitive abilities. However, somewhere in the small print it is common to find a disclaimer that says something like 'there may be extensive variations in the rate of development across domains and individuals, depending upon the person's engagement with the various domains'.[12 (p. 627)] Researchers have found positive correlations between increasing age and readiness for self-directedness.[13, 14] Interestingly, a study of 183 university students found that the older group (26 years plus) had significantly greater readiness for self-directed learning than the younger group (25 years or less).[14] This suggests that self-directedness not only develops as a person matures, but it is a personality trait that may not become apparent until many subjects have completed their formal studies. So we can assume a correlation, although not a definitive line of transition between age and maturity.

In the 1970s the idea of 'readiness' for self-directed learning took centre stage, at least for the fairly small percentage of the general population involved in researching self-directed learners. From this discussion emerged the self-directed learner's readiness scale. Developed by Guglielmino[15] in 1977, this rating scale for the self-directed learner readiness has been repeatedly subjected to investigation and has, in the main, been upheld as a valid approach. Many, many researchers have tested the scale with different demographic groups, from the more obvious student and educator groups,[13, 16, 17] to random population studies,[18] to a study assessing self-directedness during pregnancy[19] (apparently it peaks during the second trimester; certainly true for me, after the morning sickness but before I developed a significant gravitational field). Although there are some detractors from Guglielmino's model,[20] this is primarily related to the more complex applications of the scale and some methodological concerns. For a brief review of literature such as this, it is enough to look at the eight factors of self-directed learners that she identified:

1. Love of learning
2. Self-concept as an effective, independent learner
3. Tolerance of risk, ambiguity and complexity in learning
4. Creativity
5. View of learning as a lifelong, beneficial process
6. Initiative in learning
7. Self-understanding
8. Acceptance of responsibility for one's own learning

From an anecdotal viewpoint it is easy to see how many of these traits arise as an individual matures. The general increase in confidence that comes with age brings with it a greater tolerance of risk (and failure), and a broader viewpoint to encompass a vision of lifelong self-improvement. The time left behind provides greater opportunity for reflections that lead to greater self-awareness. A related alternative is the Effective Lifelong Learning Inventory (ELLI),[21] which identified seven dimensions of 'learning power'.

- Changing and learning: how deep an understanding does the learner have of themselves as a learner who evolves over time?
- Critical curiosity: how far down does the learner want to dig to understand things?
- Meaning making: how good is the learner at connecting disparate things together in a way that matters?
- Creativity: how imaginative is the learner in their personal development?
- Learning relationships: how well does the learner set up relationships to learn from and with others?
- Strategic awareness: how good is the learner's self-awareness? Of their thoughts, feelings and behaviours.
- Resilience: how long will the learner continue to persevere in the face of challenge?

The questionnaire for this tool builds up a visual, seven-spoke profile of the individual and indicates the areas that might be weakening their overall learning power. It is this learning power that dictates the effectiveness of their lifelong learning.

It is clear from the literature (and from experience) that adult educators should consider readiness for self-directed learning in terms of the level of maturity of their trainee. However, other aspects of the learner's experience and personality will also affect a trainee's readiness for self-directedness.

Professional growth

Learners in a vocational setting (like many in medical education) are likely to professionally develop in a series of fairly predictable steps. Furlong and Maynard[22] identified five stages of development for trainee teachers and it has also been applied to the GP trainee context.[23]

Early idealism

At the start of their training learners hold an ideological view of their job. They are yet to encounter the reality of the day to day job and so have a potentially unrealistic and even naïve understanding of their chosen career. Their ideas of the type of doctor/nurse/midwife they want to become are often based in their own experiences or on their perceptions drawn from TV and other media.

Survival

The Early Idealism phase is often quite short lived; reality has a tendency to quickly undermine any idealistic thoughts in the early trainee's mind. The learner is quickly overcome by the responsibility, overwhelmed by the workload and can often be found quaking and rocking silently under their desks. Joking aside, this is a vulnerable time for learners. They will need a considerable amount of support during this survival phase, their main focus will be finishing the day without doing anything to make themselves look like a total idiot. Though in many parts of medical education the stakes may be even higher with patient safety a constant concern.

Recognising the difficulties

With continued support the learner begins to see the trees: they have mastered the very basics necessary for survival, have built up the confidence to ask for help as needed and can identify more specific targets for improvement. During this phase learners need a combination of challenge and support, they need achievable targets combined with the help and guidance needed to achieve them.

Hitting the plateau

Eventually their learning will plateau; they will reach a level of competency and will be able to deal with most of the issues that arise with a degree of confidence. This is a very comfortable phase for both the learner and the educator and it is easy to allow the learner's development to halt at this point.

Moving on

This is when the learner should be motivated to take on new challenges, to push their learning into new, unexplored areas of knowledge. They may be internally or externally motivated to do this, but either way the educator needs to continue to challenge, support and guide the learner as appropriate.

In parallel with the discussion on maturity, it is important to note that different learners will pass through these stages at different rates. Additionally, the learner may revert to the Recognising the Difficulties phase after taking on a new challenge or even the Survival phase if the challenge is extreme. They will gradually hit another plateau as they develop the confidence in this new endeavour. Hopefully, they will continue to cycle through the Plateau phase to the Moving On phase and so continue to improve: a continuous cycle demonstrating self-directed learning throughout a career. Of course there are many learners in medical education that bring previous experience with them; it is important to recognise and value this experience.[24] This experience is likely to impact upon the way in which they progress through these stages of professional growth.

Consideration of the stage of professional growth may help an educator understand whether the learner is ready for self-directedness. A learner in the survival phase is unlikely to be willing or even capable of exhibiting the self-directed behaviours identified by Guglielmino.[15] A learner just hitting the plateau may be in the prime position to begin taking control of their learning.

Maturity and professional readiness

Investigate the personal readiness and professional development of the learner before embarking upon the development of self-directedness. Ensure that learners are ready to engage openly with experiences provided.

Skills, Concrete Experience (CE) 1: SD1

Baggage

We all have it. For some of us, at some points in our lives the 'baggage' we carry is hugely significant and at other times it is irrelevant, but we should always be sensitive to our learners' potential baggage. There are people who can separate themselves from their baggage and remain entirely professional, detached from their problems that are neatly segregated into compartments. Unlikely, though, isn't it? For some learners this baggage will prevent them accessing the ideals of self-directedness. Mahoney[25] identifies two different sources of baggage: externally generated and internally generated. Externally generated baggage may develop as a result of issues at work, at home or in their community. Internally generated baggage could be caused by health problems, interpersonal conflicts or more generically by their attitudes to problems and situations.

Impact of change

As well as considering the learner's baggage from their past it is worthwhile taking stock of the changes that are taking place around them in the present. With any change, at work, in training or at home, there is a period of adjustment and it is less likely that a learner will be open to self-directed learning immediately following a change.

The five stages of grief were initially proposed by Kübler-Ross[26] to describe the pattern of emotions experienced by terminally ill patients and those grieving for a loss (*see* Figure 2.1). They are now widely used as a management tool to describe the impact of change in the workplace. The principle is that people experiencing a change will be, to some extent, grieving for the prior situation. Learners may be expected to go through similar stages (reduced to three below) when any change occurs at work or at home.

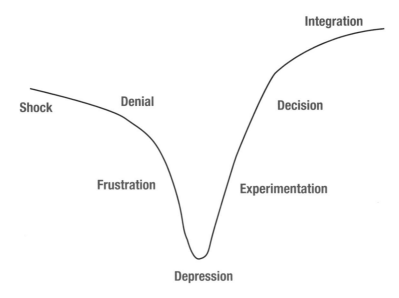

FIGURE 2.1 The five stages of grief proposed by Kübler-Ross

Stage 1

Shock, denial and frustration: during this stage individuals feel surprised and very resistant to the change, sometimes to the point of pretending that it is not happening. They will react negatively against the change and will focus on the status quo, often questioning why the change is necessary anyway.

Stage 2

Depression: in this stage the change is accepted as unavoidable, but individuals are still not engaged with the process. They may well attempt to find a scapegoat in the form of a person or organisation to blame for the inevitable change.

Stage 3

Acceptance, experimentation and integration: finally individuals recognise that the change could be for the better. They begin to look at how the change could improve their lives and try out new ways of working. At this stage people are more optimistic and enthusiastic and will finally accept the change and fully integrate it into their lives.

Attempting to engage a learner in self-directed learning during the initial stage of shock, denial and depression is likely to be unfruitful. Even if the change has nothing to do with their workplace or learning, it will still impact upon their overall engagement. An educator should be aware that a learner's readiness for self-directedness is likely to be very low during the first and second stages following a change. However, once an individual is experimenting and searching for new meaning in stage 3, they can be guided towards self-directed approaches. They could test the new system, new knowledge or skills in a self-directed manner. They could evaluate and reflect upon their learning from the change and identify the reasons for the success (or failure) of their experimentations.

Once again, different people will pass through these stages at different speeds in different situations. It is down to the skill of the educator to identify when a learner may be open to develop as a self-directed learner and when they are unlikely to engage with their learning at all effectively. The relationship between educator and learner is so important; an understanding of the learner's work life and home life will help an educator make these judgements.

Personal readiness

Ensure learners have emotional and mental space and no personal barriers that may prevent engagement with learning. They need to able to leave any personal issues to one side so that they can be motivated by a need to develop as a learner.

Motivation, Self-transcendence (ST) 1: SD2

Cultural issues

One of the criticisms of much of the research regarding self-directed learning is the lack of acknowledgment of cultural issues.[8] There is a predominance of research in European and North American societies with limited consideration of sociological factors. Research among different cultures is sporadic with no overriding conclusions. Knowles[7] points to the tensions that may exist in circumstances where the drive and the ability to be self-directed are not in sync with each other. This may well be the case if an individual feels, consciously or subconsciously, restrained by their cultural setting. Rogers and Horrocks[27] comment on this issue:

> In many societies the local culture does not encourage the development of autonomy in some groups of people (women, for instance, especially married women, in many parts of the word). Thus self-direction is partial; it may not extend to all parts of life (including education).[27] (p. 80)

Perhaps there is limited research because self-directedness is so very individual, or perhaps the issues of ethnicity are just ones that we do not feel comfortable expressing or working with.[28] There is general acceptance that cultural issues will impact on learning and on an individual's readiness for self-directed learning, but it is not easily quantifiable. Therefore judgement of the cultural issues has to fall to the skill of the educator to recognise if and when their learner is ready to be self-directed.

From cultural issues we move onto an area that provokes animated discussion: stereotyping. The uncomfortable truth is that we all draw generic conclusions and pigeon-hole information and people. It is how we deal with the vast amount of information we perceive on a daily basis. If we call it 'pattern formation' it feels more acceptable. Problems arise when the generalisations are inappropriate and it becomes a real problem if we end up unfairly labelling, making assumptions or even developing prejudices. Like it or not there are certain societal stereotypes: 'girls are not as good at maths and science' or 'Hispanic Americans or African Americans have a lower intelligence'. We may not, no, we should not hold these beliefs, but they are there and they lurk in societal memory and ignoring them will not resolve the issues. The result of lingering stereotyping is something known as stereotype threat. The stereotyped groups underperform in tests and also in ability building as a consequence of these underlying stereotypes.[29]

> Not only are stereotyped or otherwise devalued individuals unable to achieve up to their ability, stereotype threat affects individuals in learning and building abilities in the first place.[29] (p. 612)

Stereotype threat is most likely to occur when three parameters are met:

1. the learner strongly associates themselves with the group under stereotype threat
2. the learner firmly links themselves with the learning domain, and
3. the learner is very aware of the negative link between their group and their learning domain.[30]

If your learner is one of a group who suffers from stereotype threat, it may be difficult to motivate them towards our goal of self-directedness.[31] There are a number of interventions that may help combat this.[29]

- Ensure that particular groups are not given special treatment on the basis of membership to that specific group. Either positive intervention or ignoring negative behaviours can appear as special treatment. Avoid any behaviours that would communicate and emphasise a group difference.
- Values affirmation tasks – asking individuals to identify their values or most important values helps to reaffirm self-worth and integrity.
- Provide the learner with coping mechanisms to deal with the pressure of the stereotype threat. For example, by encouraging a shift in association of negative feelings from one group to another, such as not saying 'I failed because I am a black male' but 'I failed because I have recently transferred and the other trainee who transferred failed as well'. Though some caution is needed here that we do not allow them to make excuses that do not promote an action plan to pass in the future.
- Development of a growable attitude towards intelligence by, for example, asking learners to write a reflective log about the impact of relevant stereotypes.
- Develop the learner's awareness of the potential impact of stereotype threat – knowledge is power and simply knowing that they may be subject to this influence can reverse the effect.

Stereotype threat

Help learners develop an insight into the impact of stereotype threat on themselves, encourage them to find mechanisms that internally reassure them that culturally held stereotypes do not hold true for them as individuals.

Motivation, Safety (S) 1: SD3

The educator's role in readiness

So, is your learner 'ready' for self-directedness? You are best placed to make that judgement. Consider the personality traits they have exhibited thus far, the stage they have they reached in their professional growth, their cultural background, the circumstance of their studies and home life and how risk averse they appear to be. Pool all that information together and what emerges should be an indication of how far along the journey towards self-directedness your learner is to be found. The Three Pillar Model that we are constructing throughout this book will provide educators with the knowledge and skills to guide learners further down the self-directed path.

TEACHING SELF-DIRECTEDNESS

It can seem illogical to discuss the teaching of self-directedness. If self-directedness is an innate personality trait present in all adults to differing degrees as suggested by Knowles,[7] perhaps we don't need to teach it. Besides, surely it is contradictory to lead someone to self-directedness? More recently there has been a general shift in the approach to self-directedness away from the linear concept of maturation towards a view of self-directed learning as a trial and error activity. An activity in which learners make mistakes, repeat themselves, sometimes veer off course, but eventually they make progress. However, this viewpoint, taken to its extreme, also seems to deny the importance of the support provided by the educator.

It seems most likely that there is a middle ground, a balance between 'all adults are self-directed anyway' and 'self-directedness should be a series of trial and error processes'. At that balance point we find that the innate levels of self-directedness are nurtured while learners are also able to experiment in their learning. Learners need to be encouraged to take control of their own learning and given the tools and skills they need to succeed to ensure continued motivation. They must be allowed to make their own mistakes within a safe environment, to identify what works best for them as individuals. In making their own learning decisions and succeeding, they will build their confidence to try again, to take risks and tackle the fear of failure that lurks within us all. This will allow learners to develop a deeply rooted belief that they can achieve unknown goals and overcome unknown challenges. It is this combination of skills, motivation and self-belief that will develop the individual's self-directedness.

The self-directed teacher

If we wish to 'grow' (ha ha, you'll get the pun in a moment) a self-directed learner we must consider the teaching style of the teacher. Gerald Grow[1] (there it is!) identified issues in his own practice when his style of teaching and his adult students' style of learning were not congruent with each other. He borrowed from the world of situational management research to develop a model to show the importance of matching the teaching style to the readiness of the learner.

Grow's Staged Self-Directed Learner model describes four stages of learner self-direction and four corresponding stages of teaching style (*see* Table 2.1).

TABLE 2.1 The Staged Self-Directed Learner model adapted from Grow[1] (pp. 129–36)

Stage	Student	Teacher
Stage 1	*Dependent* Need explicit directions Passive learners May be systematic and thorough	*Authority* May be seen as the expert by the learner 'Pours' the knowledge into the learner
Stage 2	*Interested* Can be motivated to take part Confident See the purpose of the learning Little understanding of the teaching and learning process	*Motivator, guide* Needs to provide personal interaction and motivation Should 'sell' the learning to the learner with their enthusiasm Explains why the learner needs the knowledge and skills being taught
Stage 3	*Involved* View themselves as participants in their own learning See themselves as future equals to the teacher	*Facilitator* Share decision making Communicate with the learner about the learning taking place
Stage 4	*Self-directed* Set their own goals and standards Take responsibility for their learning	*Consultant, delegator* Still involved in learning as someone with whom learners can discuss and chart their learning Should still monitor progress

The teacher must match their style of teaching with the learner's style of learning while simultaneously encouraging the learner to move towards the next stage. A learner's stage of self-directedness may be situational; they may feel more confident undertaking some tasks than others. Therefore a teacher should be ready to identify and match their learner's needs in terms of self-directed readiness in different situations.

Brockett and Hiemstra[5] proposed the Personal Responsibility Orientation model (*see* Figure 2.2), which uses the idea discussed earlier that there are two strands to self-directedness (the learning process and the learner's personal desire for learning).

In this model they propose that self-directedness is fundamentally based upon the individual's ownership of their own thoughts and actions: their personal responsibility. From this starting point there are two aspects to consider when targeting self-direction in learning. The first, 'self-directed learning', can be considered to represent the external factors or the processes involved. It includes all aspects of the

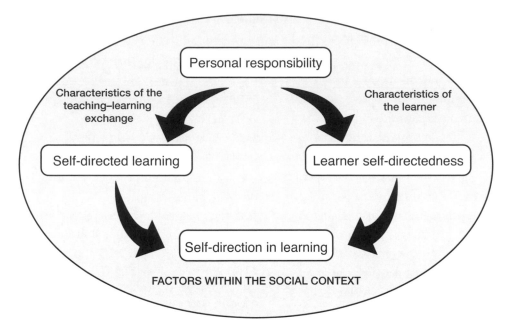

FIGURE 2.2 Personal Responsibility Orientation model by Brockett and Hiemstra

learning process such as the needs analysis, learning resources, independent study, facilitated learning, evaluation and so on. The second, 'learner self-directedness', can be considered to represent the internal factors. It is the individual learner's desire to take responsibility for their learning. Brockett and Hiemstra[4] suggest that there must be a balance between these two factors if the final goal of self-direction in learning is to be achieved. They suggest that for optimal learning the learner's desire to take responsibility must be matched by the opportunity for self-direction in the learning process. This idea of matching is obviously similar to that proposed by Grow.[1] The difference is that Brockett and Hiemstra do not suggest there should necessarily be a movement towards self-directedness. They propose that self-directedness is context specific and that this balance should be considered at each learning opportunity. Brockett and Hiemstra set this model within the wider social context, a breadth that is often left out of other considerations of self-directedness. It recognises that learners are often (usually?) part of a wider group context, they are members of teams, part of a learning organisation and/or learning network. These factors will impact upon the learning processes and their desire to take responsibility. It would be disappointing to think that we did not have any form of influence as a key part of their network. Therefore, as well as the obvious control over the learning processes, we need to have some ability to impact those internal factors that influence the learner's desire to take responsibility for their learning.

Developing a self-directed teaching programme

The previous two models by Grow[1] and Brockett and Hiemstra[5] are focused on the idea of matching teacher and learner characteristics, but they do not actually describe how to move a learner towards self-directedness. The following model by Gibbons[32] proposes a series of stages to move through when developing a self-directed programme.

1. Students thinking independently: this is the familiar teacher-directed approach, but with a gradual shift from the teacher 'telling' the students to the teacher 'asking' the students. Teachers at this stage provide guidance to students by using the learning outcomes to construct questions.
2. Teaching self-managed learning: in this second stage the students are provided with the course content but are given the time to work through it at their own pace.
3. Self-planned learning: once students are used to working through a programme independently, they can begin to decide for themselves how to complete the planned outcomes. The teacher provides learning outcomes but the learner can decide how to go about achieving them, catering to their own styles and strengths. In order to do this effectively, the student must have an understanding of their own learning.
4. Self-directed learning: at this final stage students choose their own outcomes as well as planning how to meet them.

As teachers in the adult education world we may hope that our learners are Grow stage 3 learners at least and that they already have a desire to take responsibility for their learning. This may sometimes be the case, but in other circumstances our learners need to be gradually moved on from stage 1 or 2 towards a self-directed approach. The staged model proposed by Gibbons provides an indication of how we might go about this.

A situation that treats 'the developing adult as a child to be directed what to do and what not to do will find itself faced on most occasions with major blocks to learning'.[27 (p. 80)] We must take into account the various factors discussed in the section on readiness for self-directedness. Consider their cultural background and what type of teaching and learning they have taken part in so far. Think about their home life: is their focus elsewhere for the moment and would they benefit from a period of time as a dependent learner? Grow is careful to say that a dependent learner is not necessarily a bad thing, although it is likely to limit their achievement long term. As a temporary situation it is acceptable for teaching to become a simple transfer of knowledge, as long as the teacher is working to encourage the learner's progression through the stages of self-directedness.

Self-directed teaching

Teaching strategies should shift from learners as recipients of education to learners taking control of their education. Initially this control will be within parameters (for example, outcomes or process or resources) determined by the educator, but eventually learners take full control as fully fledged self-directed learners.

Skills, Concrete Experience (CE) 2: SD4

Transformational teaching

Transformational teaching is one of the key tenets of adult learning. It involves challenging learners to understand how they have acquired the new knowledge and what their thoughts and feelings are towards the process.[33] This approach to education is a search for that transformational, 'light-bulb' moment.

Slavich and Zimbardo[33] identify five key ideas that underpin modern teaching understanding:

- active learning
- student-centred learning
- collaborative learning
- experiential learning
- problem-based learning.

There are a number of differences in these approaches, but underlying all of them is the key concept that students 'learn by doing'. Transformational teaching can happen through any of these five different approaches, but in each case there are some core theoretical underpinnings that need to be incorporated if the experiences are to be truly transformational (*see* Figure 2.3).

Transformational teaching

Provide transformational experiences for your learners, share the vision for the teaching, model the skills and knowledge, challenge and encourage your students, provide personalised feedback, plan experiential opportunities and promote reflection. This will provide high-quality, adult-orientated experiences that not only deliver high-quality learning, but also develop the learner's insight into themselves as learners.

Skills, Concrete Experience (CE) 3: SD5

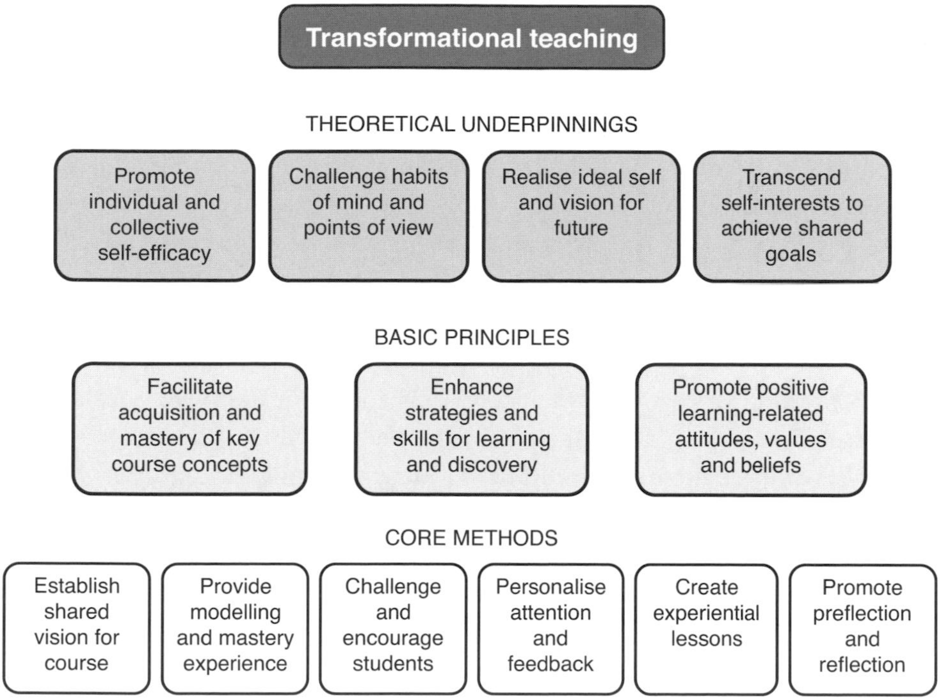

FIGURE 2.3 The theoretical underpinnings of transformational teaching as described by Slavich and Zimbardo

CHALLENGES FOR SELF-DIRECTED LEARNING

'The Curriculum'

One of the greatest challenges for self-directed learning will always be 'The Curriculum'. From the moment children enter pre-school aged three years old (or even younger), they step onto 'The Curriculum' treadmill. This is the ever changing but never-ending sequence of documents that will determine what they learn for at least the next 15 years. For those who have gone onto university courses their learning objectives have been predefined by someone else for two decades. Piskurich writes about the use of self-directed learning in business as a tool for delivering training programmes.[34] He provides an animated description of the impact of the schooling system on an individual's self-directedness.

> Most learners have one thing in common: they are not usually prepared to engage in SDL [self-directed learning]. This isn't normally due to any psychological limitation. Rather, it seems to be an acquired response to a society – and especially a school system – in which the learner is spoon fed.
>
> Babies, by way of contrast, are inherent practitioners of SDL. Few parents set

a curriculum and develop lesson plans for their newborns. Yet somehow, without such a regimented learning process, the child learns who's who, how to get food or just attention, how to walk, and, the greatest of all miracles, how to talk. … Then suddenly, this self-directed learner is thrust into schools, now learning becomes structured, there is a time for blocks, a time for puzzles, and a time for reading. … The teacher decides not only when to learn, but also what to learn and even how to learn it. … Grades, parental approval, and the chance to go to the right college replace wanting to know as the reason for learning. Self-direction disappears.[34] (p. 175)

Put into this context it is hardly surprising that adult learners don't always engage with the learning process with the level of skill and enthusiasm we feel should be associated with adults. After years of being told what to do, the freedom of a completely self-directed approach could be very disconcerting indeed. It is very easy for educators at all levels to get caught up in the delivery of the curriculum, especially when there are important (and sometimes expensive) assessments at the end of it. From a learner perspective, it is probably fair to say that the curriculum and the (inevitable) assessments weigh more heavily on their minds than does the quest for self-directedness. So it becomes a challenge for the educator to deliver the knowledge, skills and attitudes described in the curriculum in such a way that the development of self-directedness is built-in. This is just one of the delicate balancing acts educators must perform in the pursuit of the self-directed learner.

Too much self-directedness

Yes, it can happen. With many learners the challenge is getting them to take responsibility for their learning, to accept a learner led approach to tutorials, to take the initiative to find their own solutions. But there is a risk with some learners that they will become overly focused on themselves. An enthusiastic self-directed learner who constantly pursues their own interests and learning needs may do so to the detriment of their overall education. There is often, after all, a curriculum and learners must ensure their learning is relevant to external factors, like the curriculum or team requirements, as well as internal factors.

Brookfield discusses self-directed learning in the group setting where individuals must work together to achieve collective objectives and direct their learning towards common goals.[35] An individual who is too involved in their own self-directed learning may ignore these aspects of interdependence in favour of their own learning goals. So self-directedness should not be to the detriment of teamwork skills. There is that delicate balancing act again.

> ### The curriculum vs self-directedness
>
> Tread the line between curriculum requirements and self-directedness carefully to enable learners to develop in their chosen direction but also meet the requirements needed to achieve success in their programme of study.
>
> *Motivation, Self-actualisation (SA) 1: SD6*

Information overload

> In today's information-rich world, there are far more sources of information than teachers and textbooks. In fact, one could argue that students have access to too much information, much of which is contradictory, some of which is simply wrong. One of the primary goals of education then – Demetriou and his colleagues argue that it is the 'ultimate goal' – is to help students make informed, defensible judgements.'[36 (p. 16)]

The problem of information overload has been a growing issue for some time now and is a challenge that will certainly not dissipate in the future. As the Internet continues to expand filling server after server, current research will become past research that is easily accessible. Combined with the impact of social media, which gives everyone an international voice, our learners find themselves in an increasingly confusing world of information. Looking from the outside in, how do they know who the credible sources are? How do they know whether the information is valid? How can they possibly understand the overall trends, the rationale behind different sides of contentious issues when there are so many opinions available?

Herein lies one of the challenges that now face educators in developing self-directedness in their learners. This vast array of information has two sides to it: infinitely useful and indescribably important but also potentially overwhelming and daunting. Learners must pick their way through an ever expanding and sometimes (often?) contradictory collection of resources. With repetition of information not necessarily an indication of accuracy and the opportunity for every owner of a computer, tablet or smartphone to have their say, the Internet is a confusing place. We have to be aware that being technologically proficient does not necessarily mean learners have the skill to sort through this mass of information to find accurate and valid material. The risk is that when a learner does not know which way to turn, they may just switch the engine off and stop. We need to put the signpost up before they reach the junction but do it in such a way that the learner is still in charge of directing their own learning. (And we're back to the balancing act again.)

> ## Information overload
>
> Help learners negotiate their way through the vast quantity of information available, otherwise learners may abandon projects or fail to find the most relevant information. Provide them with just enough guidance to succeed but not so much that you remove their opportunity to be self-directed. Learners need to develop the skills to evaluate the validity of the information source and the tools to sieve through the information to identify relevant points.
>
> *Self-Belief, Performance Accomplishment (PA) 1: SD7*

Time

If I could find a way to bottle time and sell it in small portions I would be a billionaire. With more time I could achieve so much more: I could learn to play the piano properly, take a cake baking course and then probably spend more time at the gym to compensate. Imagine a world where you look at your daily goal list and decide that, actually, you need today to be a 27 hour day. If only. Unfortunately, I am yet to find a way to do this (maybe if I had a 27 hour day I would manage it; I think that's a paradox, though, isn't it?) so we are all stuck dealing with only 24 hours in the day. This puts pressure on how we carry out tasks. As busy educators, often the quickest way to move a conversation or learning encounter forwards is to spoon feed the learner with the information they need. Learners, meanwhile, are feeling pressured from all sides with their line manager, their patients, their partner, children or parents and their education all making demands on their precious time. The learners simply want to be told the 'quick fix' solution so that they can move on to completing the next task.

The only way to manage the challenge of time, or more specifically the lack of time, is to be conscious of it when interacting with learners. Ideally educators should ensure that tutorials are given plenty of uninterrupted time, not started late and cut short to finish early. Be aware when having even very brief conversations with the learner that you should encourage self-directedness. This is not an easy task when there is a large pile of paperwork in the inbox, but we need to try to ensure that paperwork does not become the proverbial (or literal!) barrier to developing self-directedness.

SUMMARY

If we manage to overcome these challenges and develop the self-directed learner who takes control of their own learning, identifies their own learning needs, follows them up using appropriate tools and reflects on and evaluates the outcomes, the educator can then put their feet up. Can't they? Sorry, but no, not really. As Rogers and Horrocks[27] state:

> In this process, the learner takes the initiative and plans their own structured learning process. But in most of these cases, there is some outside planner as well – someone who wrote the textbook or manual, who planned the sequence of articles in the magazines or journals used by the learner. There is still someone engaged in 'teaching' (helping the learner to learn).[27 (p. 54)]

While I'm not suggesting all educators should trot away and begin writing a text-book, there is still a place for an educator with a successfully self-directed learner. It is just that the educator's role has changed. This book does not guide the educator towards the end of the learner's development, simply towards a more collaborative process between educator and self-directed learner where the educator takes on a consulting or facilitating role rather than a teaching role. This is a model for educators to use in developing their learners into self-directed learners. While reading the rest of this book, keep your learners' individual situation in mind, and consider their readiness from all perspectives before putting in place the mechanisms suggested in the subsequent chapters.

CHAPTER 3

People and places

INTRODUCTION

Among the many things achieved by Kurt Lewin[1] (including the aforementioned experiential learning cycle) was a formula to describe behaviour: $B=f(PE)$, where B is behaviour, P is person and E is their environment. Now I do not generally get hooked by anything remotely mathsy, but there is a certain pleasing elegance to the mathematical representation that even I appreciate. In translation it means: 'behaviour is a function of both the person and their environment'. Whichever way you look at it, the meaning is clear – in order to fully understand behaviour, including learning behaviour, we have to realise that the individual (the person) and the environment (the place) are inextricably linked. So $B=f(PE)$ provides the basis for this chapter. Initially we discuss the learner as a whole and complex person, more than simply (if that can ever be said) a learner. Then we move onto the learning environment and consider how this apparently straightforward idea is far more multifaceted than we might first think.

PEOPLE

'Every man is in certain respects like all other men, like some other men and like no other men.'[2]

We continue our search for bricks to build our pillars of self-directedness by looking at the individual learner. Before we consider our learner as a learner we will take a step back and look at the learner as a whole person. Learning behaviours are obviously key to the learning process and therefore to the development of self-directedness, but there is a tendency to uncouple these learning behaviours from all other behaviours. In reality, we need to see our learners as complete entities, to consider the other aspects of their personality. As we develop our understanding of the whole person we must also encourage insight that allows the learner to understand themselves better. So we must take a two-pronged approach: (1) Develop our understanding of the learner, and (2) Work out how we will share this information with the learner so they can take it forward to impact their future learning decisions.

The Parent, Adult and Child model

There are many, (many) models of personality, including probably the most famous of all: Freud's[3] theory of id, ego and superego. However, Freud's personality model gets a little bogged down in oedipal and phallic stages that, to be honest, we probably wouldn't want to venture into with our learners. Besides, there is a certain amount of controversy over his, sometimes vague (and possibly mistranslated), conclusions, so instead we will consider the model developed by Berne as a point to begin a worthwhile examination of personality. In the 1960s Berne[4] developed a model known as Transactional Analysis in which he identified three different ego states that coexist within every individual.

> In technical language, an ego state may be described phenomenologically as a coherent system of feelings, and operationally as a set of coherent behaviour patterns. In more practical terms, it is a system of feelings accompanied by a related set of behaviour patterns. Each individual seems to have available a limited repertoire of such ego states, which are not roles but psychological realities.[4 (p. 23)]

He called the three ego states extero-psychic, neopsychic and archaeopsychic. Fortunately he went on to define them as the more easily remembered, Parent, Adult and Child states respectively. He further identified two types of Parent state: direct and indirect. When acting within the Direct Parent ego state the individual actually responds as their recognised parent model. Alternatively, in the Indirect Parent ego state the response elicited is the one that the individual believes their parents would have wanted. There are also two types of Child state: The Adaptive Child who will adapt their behaviour based upon their parents' behaviours and the Natural Child who is spontaneous and creative in their actions. Each of these states has a role to play and is important to the individual's overall personality (*see* Table 3.1). Individuals can switch between these states with varying degrees of ease and it is possible to see changes in mood, language and body language that indicate changes to the currently dominant ego state.

TABLE 3.1 The importance of Berne's ego states of Parent, Adult and Child[4]

Ego state	Type of response	Value to the overall personality
Parent state	Respond as one of our parents or as the person we believe our parents would want us to be. Our vocabulary and body language may subconsciously change to imitate our parent.	The Parent state is happy to accept that things happen in a particular way 'just because that is how it is done'. This state allows us to do things automatically, without engaging the thought processes of the Adult state, therefore saving time and energy.
Adult state	Make rational decisions based upon objective analysis of problems. Decisions made in this state are uninfluenced by the parent voice that we carry round with us.	This state provides us with significant survival mechanisms. The Adult state will risk assess and process incoming information to enable rational and detached decision making.
Child state	Responds as we would have done as a child, either adapting to parental requirements or rebelling against them. Likely to be an impulsive and poorly thought out solution. Though possibly also more creative than would be possible as Parent or Adult.	From this state we derive our enjoyment; it provides us with intuition and creativity.

This three-part model of ego states forms the basis for transactional analysis, which we will revisit in more detail later on in Chapter 4. However, in brief, transactional analysis is the idea that when we converse with someone, there is a transaction happening between the ego states involved. Our ego state response will, at least partially, depend on the other ego state in the transaction and it may change as the conversation moves onwards. Communication issues arise with certain combinations of ego states in the transaction.

As with many of the ideas in this chapter (and indeed in the whole book), one of the most important and useful actions using this concept is to share it with the learner. Development of self-directedness for future contexts requires insight into their own behaviours. If learners can begin to recognise their own ego states, they can develop a better insight into their own behaviours. They could even begin to realise when they are behaving in accordance with a particular ego state and adapt accordingly. It is likely that a learner who is experiencing a heightened sense of emotional arousal, that is high levels of stress and anxiety, will find their ego state dominated by the child. An individual who can recognise this in themselves and concentrate on shifting into their adult state may find they can approach a situation more rationally.

> ### Berne's[4] ego states
>
> Allow your learner to develop an understanding of Berne's ego states and recognise them in themselves. Achievement of self-awareness with regards to their ego states will allow them to recognise when their child ego state is in control, with this understanding they may be able to better control their emotions in stressful situations.
>
> *Self-belief, Emotional Arousal (EA) 1: PP1*

Personality

Psychologists could stay up late into the night discussing the validity of categorising personality types. Can all human beings be pigeon-holed into a fixed number of different categories? Do you act as the same person in all circumstances? Has your personality remained unchanged for the last 10 years? Hmmm. Questions for another discussion.

There is, however, a general consensus of the 'Big Five' personality factors:[5] neuroticism, extraversion, openness, agreeableness, conscientiousness.

- Neuroticism: the tendency to be depressed, anxious, insecure, vulnerable and hostile
- Extraversion: the tendency to be sociable and assertive and to have positive energy
- Openness: the tendency to be informed, creative, insightful and curious
- Agreeableness: the tendency to be accepting, conforming, trusting and nurturing
- Conscientiousness: the tendency to be thorough, organised, controlled, dependable and decisive.[5 (p. 22)]

There is much research into personality from a continuum viewpoint as well. One of the more enduring theories is that of Eysenck,[6] who identified two main and two additional dimensions of personality:
- Main:
  - Neuroticism ↔ Emotional stability
  - Extraversion ↔ Introversion
- Additional:
  - Low intelligence ↔ High intelligence
  - Normal ↔ Psychotic

The first three of these are seen to have a mathematically normal distribution with the fourth, psychoticism, having an asymmetrical distribution. It should be acknowledged that the last of these personality dimensions has been controversial: not everyone accepts that 'us normal folk' only differ by degrees from psychotic individuals. But (hopefully) we do not usually have to deal with psychotic trainees.

Whether we accept a categorising or a continuum-based approach to personalities, pigeon-holing is how our minds deal with enormous amount of information we receive on a daily basis. Our brain simply decides that it has seen a similar situation before and uses that situation to make predictions about the current context. Since we are instinctively categorising in our pattern recognition processes, it seems reasonable to utilise a model that helps to do this for personality types. We could take all personality traits and place ourselves somewhere along a scale from 0 to 100, but this would become ridiculously unwieldy. So personality 'tests' take a handful of traits that are general enough to be useful. Possibly the most well-known is the Myers-Briggs[7] personality inventory, a four-dimensional analysis of personality based on the original work by Carl Jung in the early 1920s. The personality traits are based upon the concept that people vary in how they perceive information and how they form judgements based on this information. Essentially there are four continuums and every individual will exhibit preferences of varying strengths for each one (*see* Table 3.2).

TABLE 3.2 Myers-Briggs dimensions of personality[7]

Extraversion (E)	Focus on information from the external world	Introversion (I)	Focus on information from their own internal world
Sensing (S)	Focus on the pure facts, the basic information provided	Intuition (N)	Prefer to interpret the information and add meaning to it
Thinking (T)	The focus of decision making is on the logical process	Feeling (F)	The focus of decision making is on the people involved and the individual circumstances
Judging (J)	When decision making involves the outside world the focus is on getting the decision made and making things happen	Perceiving (P)	The focus is more open to new information and new options that might arise from the outside world

Once a preference for each continuum has been established individuals can be grouped into one of 16 possible combinations, such as ENTJ or ISTP. The test is actually more sensitive than this and will provide a strength of preference (e.g. a strong preference for Extraversion with a moderate preference for Intuition and so on), generally though the four letter code, with the 16 possible categories, proves complex enough for most contexts.

In terms of self-directedness this is a useful tool to help learners understand themselves as part of the learning process. As they reflect on their experiences they should be able to place their thoughts within an understanding of their own preferences, how they perceive information and their tendencies when forming judgements and making decisions.

Personality types

Encourage your learners to identify personality types such as the Myers-Briggs[7] personality inventory and openly discuss the implications of the findings. The increased self-awareness and insight will provide them with an internal context to consider their reflections, improving the level of insight into their learning needs.

Skills, Reflective Observation (RO) 1: PP2

Intelligence

Goleman[8] identifies three domains of excellence: raw intelligence (IQ), emotional intelligence (EQ) and expertise. For my first trick I will dispense with the idea of expertise – this relates to practical skills and the ability to apply knowledge in everyday and exceptional circumstances. Trainees will be developing these curriculum-related skills throughout their training. From the perspective of self-directedness this expertise is found in our Skills Pillar. Therefore, much of this book will be studying the development of the expertise for self-directedness and we shall not look at it further at this juncture. I am also going to be a chicken and omit a discussion of intelligence. This is a hazardous area of nature versus nurture literature and an ethical minefield for researchers and educators. It is obvious that we must consider the potential of our individual learner, but far be it from me to decide where the origins of that potential lie. In Chapter 6 we will consider how best to identify and support learners of different abilities, but a discussion of intelligence theory at this point is likely to be unfruitful and potentially provocative. I will, in a later section, make a brief exception to explore the related idea of fixed and growable attitudes towards intelligence.

So, having successfully ducked two of Goleman's domains of excellence, that only leaves us with the third to discuss in further detail at this point. The significance of emotional intelligence in relation to a raw intelligence quotient is a continuing area of research and discourse, and I am not going to make a case for the importance of one versus the other. However, it would be naïve to ignore the idea of emotional maturity and emotional intelligence when attempting to develop self-directedness.

Emotional intelligence can be defined as 'the capacity for recognising our own feelings and those of others, for motivating ourselves and for managing emotions well in ourselves and in our relationships'.[8] (p. 317) and also as 'problem solving with and about emotions'.[9] (p. 97)

Additional detail about the concept is provided by the five basic competencies described by Goleman.[8]

- Self-awareness: Knowing what we are feeling in the moment
- Self-regulation: Handling our emotions
- Motivation: Using our deepest preferences to move and guide us towards our goals
- Empathy: Sensing what people are feeling, being able to take their perspective; and cultivating rapport and attunement with a broad diversity of people
- Social skills: Handling emotions in relationships well and accurately reading social situations.[8] (adapted from p. 318)

Or alternatively by the four branches devised by Mayer *et al.*[9]

- Perceiving emotion accurately
- Using emotion to facilitate thought
- Understanding emotion
- Managing emotion.[9] (p. 97)

In general there are two aspects to consider, first, understanding your own feelings: self-awareness, using your own emotions positively, an inward-facing attribute. Second, perceiving and understanding the feelings of others: empathy, an outward-facing attribute. In either case we can consider how effectively we, and our learners, are able to solve emotional problems.

Emotional intelligence

Develop learner insight into their emotional intelligence. A greater understanding of their strengths and weaknesses with regard to their own self-awareness, self-regulation, motivations, empathy and social skills will allow them to reflect more deeply on their involvement and perceptions.

Skills, Reflective Observation (RO) 2: PP3

Empathy and understanding

Development of emotional intelligence and an individual's insight into their emotional intelligence will help them to form stronger supportive bonds with those around them.

Motivation, Belongingness (B) 1: PP4

Creativity

Alongside this discussion of expertise, raw intelligence and emotional intelligence is creativity. The consideration of creativity may seem unusual, but the common usage of 'creativity' can most certainly be broadened to include the inventiveness needed to develop new ideas, to problem solve and in our context to abstractly contextualise new information. If we consider any group of people that we work with, it is immediately obvious that some are better at producing the original solution than others; these people are often called divergent thinkers. Learners who are more accomplished divergent thinkers are more likely to be able to suggest successful ways in which to meet their own learning needs.

So the next question is obviously: how on Earth can you measure creativity? This is a shaky area of research, and some have tried to quantify idea generation through structured thinking processes (e.g. Toubia[10]) while others have generated test questions to determine levels of divergent thinking.

> All ask the testee to think of lots of answers to a question, not just one. Questions might be: How many uses can you think of for a brick, or a paperclip? Or: If gravity were suddenly to cease, what would be some of the consequences? Answers can be scored for fluency, which is the number of answers produced, and for flexibility, which is the number of shifts from one sort of use to another. Answers to the paperclip question such as to clean out your ears, to clean your nails, to pick your nose and to clean your navel would get a reasonably high score for fluency but not for flexibility. An answer which went: to clean your nails, to make a fuse, a propeller for a model aircraft, a pipe cleaner and an ear-ring for a punk – would get a higher score for flexibility.[11] (p. 43)

There are a number of issues: first the link between divergent thinking and creativity is not firmly proved. Second, the strength of the link between creativity and real life problem solving is also not clearly defined. Third, there is a question over whether there is a significant difference between divergent thinking and IQ. Given all these problems it is perhaps unwise to go too far in our use of this area of research, but it is significant to our consideration of self-directedness. It is pretty common for learners, upon identifying a learning need, to suggest the means to meet this need is 'I will read up about it'. Conversely, there are those who decide to sit in a clinic, take an e-module, arrange a meeting with a specialist, focus future workplace-based assessments on the learning need, organise a learning set to reinforce and develop new knowledge, and ask peers to role model patients with similar complexities. While both these types of learner may exhibit self-directedness, the latter is more likely to have repeated successful and positive learning experiences and therefore is more likely to continue the learning process into their future careers.

Biggs[12] states that 'genuine creativity requires significant, substantive knowledge in a given area'.[12 (p. 66)] So how to develop the learner's ability to think creatively when it comes to meeting their own learning needs? The self-directed learner will be able to consider alternative solutions and evaluate the potential outcomes because they will have substantive knowledge of the possible options available to them. We can make creative learning suggestions that learners may be able to apply to future similar circumstances. This may not directly influence their fundamental creativity, but it will increase the tools available to them when approaching a learning need. They will demonstrate creativity when it comes to applying the previously used methods to a new learning need. We can also be less forward about it and encourage the learner to make suggestions themselves using probing questions. The most effective approach will depend upon the natural creativity of your learner.

Creativity

Develop the learner's ability to think creatively about the potential solutions to a learning need. Use questioning to elicit novel approaches from learners and provide plentiful examples of tools or approaches that learners could apply to future learning needs.

Skills: Abstract Conceptualisation (AC) 1: PP5

The stress test

Stress. A sticky and ethically grey area for research; a serious problem for employers everywhere; and a major headache for the Secretary of State for Work and Pensions as he (or she) tries to make the benefits books balance. Some would rather that the whole idea of 'stress' is left unspoken, but it can quickly become a large grey mammal in the room if we don't talk about it. So let's just say it. We are all vulnerable to stress; some people get more stressed than others and some people get stressed more often than others. A stressed individual is unlikely to respond well to the suggestions in this book, so we must be alert to our learner's level of stress and also to their ability to deal with stress.

The Social Readjustment Ratings Scale (SRRS) is not (as it sounds) a State-provided tool in some fictional, dictatorial future. It is a scale produced by Holmes and Rahe,[13] two doctors, for using major life events as a predictor for ill health. They questioned their patients to determine what significant life events had happened to each of them in the 12 months preceding their illness. The outcome was a list of 40 plus major events, such as divorce, death (of friends and families of course; death of the learner would probably put an end to the drive for self-directedness), pregnancy, changes to work and home life. Even things like Christmas made it onto this list. Each was given a numerical value with the intention being that individuals could calculate their own likelihood of developing a stress-related illness.

It is unnecessary to replicate the whole list here because our model of self-directedness is about the individual learner and from this perspective there is a significant flaw in the SRRS: it assumes all individuals will experience a change in the same way. This is too simplistic; there is such a thing as an amicable divorce, stressful certainly but not as stressful as a drawn out battle for custody of children. By all means keep these things in mind when considering your learner's drive for self-directedness; as was discussed in Chapter 2, learners need to be ready for self-directedness and part of this is considering the changes happening around them.

The second issue with the SRRS is that these are major life events that will happen rarely if ever for some people. My husband will be pleased to see in print that I have no intentions of filing for divorce. Kanner *et al.*[14] developed a tool entitled The Hassles Scale, the origin of the scale being that stress is derived from the small but cumulative day to day events that hassle us. For example, losing our car keys (darling daughter left them jammed in the conservatory door), things getting more expensive (the research may be 30 years old but, still, how very current), physical appearances (I may be a mother of two but I still manage to get a spot on the end of my nose before any (rare) evening out). These little hassles are cumulative in nature and can be dissipated by a strong network of support. Different individuals will deal with them with varying success, but there is evidence of a significant link between the number and severity of hassles such as these and serious stress illnesses such as depression and anxiety.

So what can we do about it? There are two obvious roles for an educator in helping learners minimise stress. First, we can work, as much as is possible and sensible, to remove unnecessary hassles from their learning environment. Second, we can be part of the support network that helps to dissipate the impact of hassles over which the learner has no control. Most likely, this will simply be lending an ear on the bad days. This is important in the context of our Self-belief Pillar, as the level of emotional arousal being experienced by an individual will affect their self-efficacy. A stressed learner is unlikely to have the self-belief to make full and sustained attempts at achieving new things.

Stress and hassles

Where possible remove the small, unnecessary hassles for learners and develop their ability to recognise and manage the impact of small hassles. Take the time to listen to your learner's moans; they may be small and apparently insignificant 'hassles', but the cumulative effect can be significant in the learner's ability to engage with a drive for self-directedness.

Self-belief, Emotional Arousal (EA) 2: PP6

Learning styles

Having now considered some of the wider aspects of personality, we will focus on the learning behaviours that form the basis for many of the interactions between teacher and learner. There are a number of different ways to categorise learning types and styles, in fact there are now so many that some researchers have started trying to bring them together to meta-analyse learning styles of the individual (e.g. Goulding and Syed-Khuzzan[15]). We shall take a look at a few of the most well-known.

Learning types are certainly a useful way to group types of learners, but we should be a little cautious because (similarly to personality types) the learning styles of all of humankind cannot really be classified into four categories. There are a significant number of educationalists who believe that learning styles are at best unhelpful and at worst destructive. Ever the compromiser, though, I prefer to take a middle ground and see both the value in the conversation as well as the need to step back and take all labels with a pinch of metaphorical salt.

The VARK model

Fleming and Mills[16] developed the VARK model of learning preferences with an underlying principle that the information has to be shared with the learner. They produced a questionnaire that allows learners and their educators to determine the teaching strategies that will be most effective for each individual. The focus of their modal preferences questionnaire is 'as a catalyst to empower students to reflect on their own sensory preferences and modify their study methods accordingly'.[16 (p. 137)] Fleming and Mills found, by questioning students, that many of them believed that the root cause of their difficulties in learning was the manner in which the knowledge was presented, whether orally, written, graphically or through concrete experiences. Following these conversations they developed a simple questionnaire that can be used to identify the perceptual mode through which individuals learn best.

- Visual (V): Preference for graphical and symbolic ways of representing information.
- Aural (A): Preference for 'heard' information (i.e. lectures, tutorials and discussions).
- Read/Write (R): Preference for information printed as words.
- Kinaesthetic (K): Preference related to the use of experience and practice (simulated or real).[16] (adapted from p. 140)

Although Visual and Read/Write are both visual it is more practical to divide them into graphical and written. The kinaesthetic preference provides a few difficulties for categorisation because the experience used to convey the knowledge could utilise visual, read/write or aural means. Therefore, this mode takes preference when classifying a task with the means of conveyance being a secondary consideration.

Learners are encouraged to answer questions with the answer that best suits their likely response; they can select more than one answer for a particular question. The questions provide specific but universal experiences to elicit people's preferred responses and therefore their preferred learning style.

1. You are about to give directions to a person. She is staying in a hotel in town and wants to visit your house. She has a rental car. Would you:
   V) Draw a map on paper?
   A) Tell her the directions?
   R) Write down the directions (without a map)?
   K) Collect her from the hotel in your car?

8. Which of these games do you prefer?
   V) Pictionary
   R) Scrabble
   K) Charades

12. A new movie has arrived in town. What would most influence your decision to go (or not go)?
    A) Friends talked about it.
    R) You read a review about it.
    V) You saw a preview of it.[16] (pp. 150–1)

The outcome of the questionnaire will identify one or two preferences that can serve as a stimulus for discussion with the learners.

The most realistic approach to accommodation of learning styles in teaching programs should involve empowering students through knowledge of their own learning styles to adjust their learning behaviour to the learning programs they encounter.[16 (p. 138)]

Honey and Mumford

An alternative model for considering learning styles was devised by Honey and Mumford,[17] based upon Kolb's Experiential Learning Cycle[18] (*see* Figure 3.1). Honey and Mumford used Kolb's learning cycle to derive and label four learning types and developed a questionnaire to help identify four learner styles.

- Activist: those who learn by doing, very active individuals who prefer immediate action and will want to try things out.
- Reflector: those who like to spend time observing and considering all the options available before approaching new tasks.
- Theorist: those who like theories and logical processes, they will prefer to have a model to structure new ideas.
- Pragmatist: those who will want to know the why and the how, very practical in their approach and like to work with real-life situations.

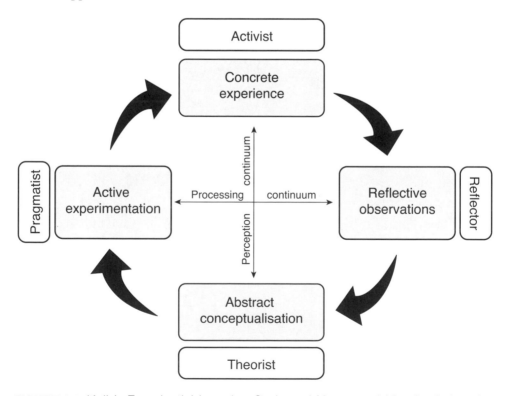

FIGURE 3.1 Kolb's Experiential Learning Cycle and Honey and Mumford's learning preferences

It is likely that an individual will have a strong preference for one or two of these with weaker preferences for the others. This information can be used to build appropriate teaching plans and use suitable strategies to meet the preferred styles; however, it is also important to develop the learners' weaker styles. This is particularly relevant in our context of developing self-directedness by building the learning Skills Pillar. We used Kolb's Experiential Learning Cycle to structure this pillar and we need our learners to have the skills for all four stages of the learning process if we are to help them be self-directed. On that basis, while the Honey and Mumford learning styles offer us interesting insight into our learners (and one that we should share with our learners), it does not really provide us with a specific brick for our Skills Pillar. The questionnaire is very useful to demonstrate to us the starting point of our learners' learning skills. It will allow us to work out which particular skills bricks we will need to focus on to successfully build the Skills Pillar of self-directedness for our specific learner. We need to find how to develop all of the learning styles in our learners, irrespective of their initial preference, to ensure that their success in their learning pursuits.

> ### Learning styles
>
> Use learning styles (such as VARK,[16] Honey and Mumford[17]) to plan for effective learning experiences for your learner – balance need to make the material accessible for your learner with the development of alternative styles. Once the learner has insight into their learning preferences they will also be able to plan effective learning experiences for themselves.
>
> *Skills, Concrete Experience (CE) 4: PP7*

Houle's types of learner

Houle[19] identified three types of motivation for adult learners, and although motivation will be discussed further in Chapter 7 it is worth considering the natural position of your learner with regard to lifelong learning.

- Goal-orientated learners: these learners will take part in learning in order to achieve a particular objective. To become self-directed these learners will have to learn to identify specific aims when they embark on a learning process so that they have something to work towards.
- Activity-orientated learners: these learners take part in learning because they enjoy the process. They may like to have the opportunity to meet and work or socialise with people outside their usual workplace or want something to do in the evenings other than trashy television. If your learner is motivated for

these reasons they need to specifically identify it. A learner who is motivated by working in groups would likely find it difficult to complete an individual, online e-module.

- Learning-orientated learners: these learners like learning for the sake of learning. They are the easiest to motivate to be self-directed, though they can lose focus if they feel the learning is not valuable, and their broad interests mean they can easily decide to go and learn something else.

When we think about the Maslow stage of self-actualisation we usually consider the content of the learning: the artist who 'must' paint may find learning a new medium very self-actualising. What we don't often consider is how the learning process itself can be self-actualising. We can use Houle's types of learners to tap into these motivations. If a learner is going to be fulfilled by achieving a goal, by working with others or by acquiring new knowledge they can utilise this to ensure they set themselves up to be fully satisfied by their learning experience.

Type of learner

Uncover the natural standpoint of your learner with regard to lifelong learning. Find out if they are goal orientated, activity orientated or learning orientated. Ensure your learner has insight into this aspect of their personality to increase their awareness of their own motivations and allow them to make learning opportunities a rewarding and self-actualising experience.

Motivation, Self-Actualisation (SA) 2: PP8

The Educator

Learning styles

It is common for discussions regarding the people in education to revolve around the learner. We tend to forget that there are two sides to the learning relationship and, in fact, we need to include the educator in Lewin's[1] equation: perhaps $B=f(PE)$ where P = Teacher + Learner.

Educators should reflect upon their own learning styles and preferences and consider the impact this might have on the learner. If your learning style is activist how would a reflector feel in a learning environment created by you? If you naturally learn through written information are you able to cater for those who learn graphically or aurally? It can be useful to pool ideas with other educators with different learning styles to find out how they might approach different learning encounters.

Fixed or growable intelligence?

The educator's attitude towards potential – whether explicit or implicit – will inevitably impact upon the learner's achievements and the educator's judgements. It has been found that while explicit attitudes are likely to be positive, implicit attitudes are more likely to be negative.[20] So having previously ducked the issue of intelligence, this section is the closest that I will get with a look at attitudes towards intelligence. There are two opposing approaches to education:[21] those that believe intelligence is fixed and those that believe it is growable, and it is worth taking time to reflect on your own standpoint. Do you believe that intelligence is fixed, that it is a predetermined personality parameter that cannot be altered? Or do you believe that intelligence is something that can grow and increase with the right learning opportunities and the right environment? We know now that the brain can continue adapting and making new connections throughout adulthood, but how far do you believe this translates into an unlimited intelligence?

This is a controversial area of research, particularly if you enter the field of the education of gifted children. 'The Bell Curve'[22] is a good example of the controversy that research like this can cause: research that suggested rigid links between intelligence and many factors including, most controversially, race. There are many who believe that giftedness is a given personality trait, but there are equally many who believe that anyone can be gifted at a subject if they work hard enough. If you believe that intelligence is fixed and predetermined this will impact upon your approach to your learner and, explicit or not, it is likely they will pick up on an attitude that might imply they cannot learn a particular complex idea. With an attitude of growable intelligence your learner will pick up on the idea that if they apply themselves correctly they can achieve. The latter attitude will encourage them to believe that they can succeed if they work both hard and smart.

Growable intelligence

Consider your own attitude towards intelligence: fixed or growable. Work towards approaching your learners with a mindset of growable intelligence, when learners believe that you have an open attitude towards their potential they are more likely to take on board your encouragements.

Self-belief, Verbal Persuasion (VP) 1: PP9

Educator credibility

The reflective skills of the educator are not just important with regards to attitude towards intelligence. Educators need to look carefully at how all aspects of their approach impact on the developing relationship with their learner. Self-directedness will be best nurtured within a trusting relationship. This means the learner has to trust that their teacher has the skills and knowledge to teach them but also trust that they have the right personal qualities and have the learner's best interests at heart. Brookfield[23] describes the authenticity of the teacher as consisting of six aspects:

1. Being explicit about how the teaching and learning experience is to be organised and the evaluative criteria used.
2. Making sure one's words and actions as an instructor are consistent and congruent.
3. Being ready to admit errors.
4. Revealing aspects of oneself as a person outside an instructor's role.
5. Taking students seriously by listening carefully to their concerns, anxieties or problems.
6. Realising the power of role modelling.

The credibility of the educator is important for the development of self-directedness because we need the learner to trust the encouragement of the educator. When building our third pillar, self-belief, verbal persuasion will be an important tool. In addition to outwardly demonstrating a belief in the growable intelligence of the learner, it is important to build wider credibility by following through and being authentic in our dealings with learners.

Credibility

It is important that educators are credible role models; the learners need to believe in their authenticity. Educators should strive to be clear and explicit, make sure their words and actions are congruent, be willing to admit mistakes and be open and receptive. This will increase the level of trust and therefore increase the impact of encouragement.

Self-belief, Verbal Persuasion (VP) 2: PP10

PLACES

When I first think of the learning environment I see classrooms with plastic chairs and two-person tables in rows, or (if the teacher was really cool) in groups of three so six of us could sit round the table. As I mentally drift through my own education I move from these classrooms into lecture theatres where I sat squeezed behind long 'desks' and squashed up against other students in a shared blur of boredom and hangover. The common theme in these is the tables and chairs and it is probably inevitable that consideration of the place of learning begins in the physical world.

However, it is also much more than this, as the learning environment expands beyond the physical tables and chairs to the psychological and emotional aspects that define the general ambience of a place of learning. Hiemstra,[24] who has devoted much of his career to researching and improving learning environments, defines the learning environment as 'all of the physical surrounding, psychological or emotional conditions, and social or cultural influences affecting the growth and development of an adult engaged in an educational enterprise'.[24 (p. 8)] In addition, the modern learning environment also has to embrace the virtual world, as we need to consider how the virtual environment supports our learners and helps them become more self-directed.

Therefore, this section is divided into three subsections: the physical environment, the virtual environment and the general ambience. We will consider research in each area and uncover some of the bricks needed to build our pillars and, in doing so, find the things we can do as educators to develop self-directedness.

The physical environment and learning types

We have already discussed how learning types can be important in our consideration of the individual person, whether that is the learner or the educator. It is also something to keep in mind when devising the physical learning environment. Visual learners will appreciate colourful displays, aural learners may like background music to aid their recall, kinaesthetic learners may appreciate space for role play or video replay equipment. A reflector may prefer a quiet room, with the opportunity for one to one conversations or even time alone. On the other hand, an activist may want the opportunity to try things out immediately so perhaps it would be useful to have whiteboards or flip charts for immediate brainstorming. This is all about making the learning experience useful and relevant in terms of learning preferences. The more positive and useful we can make these experiences, the more likely it is that our learners will be open to future experiences.

The learning environment

Once your learner has insight into their own learning preferences discuss the sort of physical environment they might like in relation to their learning preference in order to maximise the impact of the learning experience. This may vary depending on the nature of the topic so it is worth revisiting on a regular basis.

Skills, Concrete Experience (CE) 5: PP11

The SPATIAL model

In considering the physical aspects of the environment the SPATIAL model developed by Fulton[25] (how long did he work to get that acronym?) is a useful starting point. His basic concerns regarding research into this area of education were that research tended to be compartmentalised into one area, such as architectural research, psychological research, sociological research and so on. The SPATIAL model is intended to bring these together and to ensure that consideration of the physical environment is set against the impact on learning behaviours not just behaviour generally (*see* Table 3.3).

TABLE 3.3 The three levels of the SPATIAL model for learning environment[25]

Satisfaction **P**articipation **A**chievement	The physical environment can affect the learner's level of satisfaction, level of participation and overall achievement.
Transcendent attributes **I**mmanent attributes	The importance of perception in considering those factors that lie out of the learner's control. The learner's perception of these can be very subjective.
Authority **L**ayout	External realities that can be changed by altering the physical set-up of the room.

It is interesting to note how heavily the learner's perceptions are considered in this model. Fulton[25] identifies two important ways of defining the physical environment – the material attributes and the perceived effect. He provides the example of the number of people in a room: when considering this in a purely material manner we could discuss the density of the room, the number of people per square metre, and make a decision on a reasonable numerical value. However, this mathematical approach to the density of people in a room would not account for the perception of crowding by different individuals. Different cultures and different individuals have varying tolerances for personal space that will impact how they perceive the learning environment. What might work for one group of learners may feel tense and overcrowded for another. This may also depend on whether the learners know one another, as personal space adjusts as we get to know people. What this demonstrates is that there is not a one size fits all solution to physical space. Consider the twice yearly duvet swap argument between me and my husband: the air temperature is the same on both sides of the bed but every spring and autumn we fail to agree on the date to decrease or increase the tog rating.

So let's look a little closer at this model. The first of the three levels (Satisfaction, Participation and Achievement) are the three factors that provide a three-dimensional definition of learning. The physical space provided can impact upon all three of these factors and the effects may work together or they may contradict one another. For example, a formal classroom layout could improve achievement but reduce satisfaction. So this first level is about how we might measure the impact of changes to the physical environment.

This three-dimensional measurement of learning is set against the second layer which describes the impact of perception. The model describes two aspects: those factors that often transcend the learner's control, such as temperature, lighting, noise levels, crowding and the way these factors are internally processed. Fulton suggests that educators can address these issues firstly by making it possible to alter the physical attributes and secondly by encouraging the learner to visualise the space they are working in and how they perceive it. This is congruent with the idea that to develop self-directedness we have to achieve two things: we have to encourage our learners to be self-directed in the immediate learning situation but also develop their skills for self-directedness in the future. A significant part of this latter aim is the development of the learner's insight into themselves as a learner.

The second level also begins to clarify the need, wherever possible, for an individualised approach to the physical layout. For example, in a more formalised classroom setting some learners may be less satisfied with the approach whereas others may actually be more satisfied as they find they are able to avoid participation by isolating themselves to one side of the room. It all comes down to the perception of the individual learner.

The final level is the two interrelated factors of authority and layout. Fulton explains that the two are closely linked because the layout of the room and ability to make changes to it are indicative of the locus of the authority in the room. The layout can be used to shift power from the educator to the learner.

Fulton suggests a series of questions for educators to use when assessing the physical learning environment they are providing.

Satisfaction, Participation and Achievement
1. Have learners been asked how satisfied they are with the space being used?
2. Have distracting physical features been removed or eliminated whenever possible?
3. Do learners stay on task in the setting that is provided?
4. Does body language indicate a desire to leave?
5. Does the place allow learners to use appropriate learning strategies?
6. Can auditory, tactile and visual learning styles be used?

Transcendent and Immanent
7. Are the location and room size appropriate for the planned learning activities?
8. Do the furnishings 'fit' the people who will be using them?

9. What messages about learning could be assumed by the learners from the conditions of the space?

10. Is there potential for some individuals to be challenged or offended by some aspect of the space?

Authority and Layout

11. Can changes be made in the learning environment?

12. Who can make changes?

13. Does the space meet minimal safety and comfort standards?

14. Are necessary special requirements such as appropriate audio-visual equipment available?[25 (p. 21)]

To support development of self-directedness we need to, as much as is possible, hand over control of the physical environment to our learners. Through discussion, develop the learner's understanding of their own needs and preferences and give them the control to meet them.

- What type of physical learning environment do they need to maximise their own satisfaction, participation and achievement?
- How do they perceive the factors that are out of their control?
- Consider the different learning environments they have worked in: what were their own satisfaction levels, their participation levels and how well did they achieve in each scenario? Identify any specific distractions or problems in each learning environment.
- Consider situations where the different dimensions conflict with each other and discuss the reasons for this to help develop insight.

Learner environmental control

Discuss your learner's preferences for the physical environment and how successfully they have learned in different environments previously.

Motivation, Physiological (P) 1: PP12

The third layer also provides a further consideration: in developing self-directedness we want our learners to take control, to develop independence, so perhaps this should start at the very basic level of the physical environment. Give them some control over the physical environment and the locus of authority and power begins to shift towards the learner. Increasing the learner's perceived control within the learning environment will help improve their self-confidence in their learning.

Physical locus of authority

When setting up a room for a learning encounter, consider the locus of authority. Will the learner feel powerless in this learning situation or feel that they have a degree of control over the learning encounter? Increased learner authority in the layout will develop their sense of responsibility for their learning process and the increased self-esteem that goes with increased responsibility.

Motivation, Self-esteem (SE) 1: PP13

The physical environment for feedback

The SPATIAL model provides an excellent model to consider a multitude of different learning scenarios. In medical education (as in most environments) it is not always possible to provide the perfect learning environment, but that does not have to stop us working towards it. There is a very specific type of learning scenario that is common in medical education: individual feedback, reviews or workplace assessments. In these circumstances the above ideas will still all apply, but there are a couple of other things to take into account. Starr,[26] in her book on coaching skills, provides a few questions to be considered when beginning a coaching conversation. However, they apply to any form of more private learning encounter when a learner may feel exposed and vulnerable in the discussion.

1. Is your room quiet enough?
2. Are the chairs in the room comfortable but not 'cosy'? (You want to stay awake.)
3. Is the room private, i.e. away from other people's hearing, out of view etc?
4. Can you sit where you can see and hear your coachee properly?
5. Is your coachee happy and comfortable with the room?'[26 (p. 125)]

None of this is rocket science, but if a learner is being given feedback or being expected to expose areas of weakness through discussion they need to feel secure in their learning environment. It can be all too easy to end up having these conversations behind curtains or with doors propped open without thinking about the learner perspective. The development of self-directedness has to go hand in hand with the development of insight. This can be done through clever conversational questioning, but it will only work if the learner feels they are in a safe environment.

Feedback environment

When giving feedback or expecting your learner to expose areas of weakness in some way, ensure the learning environment is safe and secure, away from perceived prying ears. This will fulfil the learner's security needs and allow them to develop the necessary skills to identify their own learning needs in the future.

Motivation, Safety (S) 2: PP14

The virtual environment

So now we move from the physical world to the virtual world. Modern healthcare is becoming increasingly computer driven and there is no avoiding the fact that the accessibility and availability of intranet and Internet resources is going to impact upon our learners' experience. However, research that can be applied to the self-directedness movement is scant. There is growing research on Computer Based Learning Environments: things like virtual learning environments (VLEs) and online e-modules and so on, but much of this is not overly relevant to the medical educator working at the front line. However, we will cherry pick a few useful points that indicate how to best utilise and organise the virtual aspects of learning that fall within our control.

Virtual learning environments are becoming increasingly widespread in educational institutions from primary schools to universities. These allow learners remote access to learning opportunities and increasingly allow learners to submit work online. For the majority of healthcare learning, these VLEs will be too complicated and expensive to be useful. However, there are some useful lessons to draw from evaluations of VLE use. In 2009 OFSTED[27] carried out an evaluation of VLE use and found that 'The best VLEs reviewed allowed learners to reinforce their routine work, or catch up on missed lessons. In those best cases the material offered was fun and helpful and was being used well by learners. In the least effective examples, documents had been dumped on the system and forgotten.'[27] (p. 4) Notice the implied reference to self-directedness here: allowing learners to catch up on missed work or take time to reinforce new information. We should not be expecting our learners to miraculously develop all the skills needed to be self-directed overnight. Like any other skill set, we need to approach it in small sections and provide the support and challenge necessary for diverse learners. 'Providing students with a high amount of learner control works well for students who are highly self-regulated and not so well for those who are not.'[28] (p. 441)

With this in mind, once learners have an identified learning goal, we can nudge them towards suitable resources, if these are available online or on an intranet it will be an easier task for the learner to work towards meeting this learning need. For this stage of skill development we have effectively removed the need to hunt for the correct resources and therefore minimised the risk of the learner losing focus and never meeting their identified learning need.

Virtual resources

Build up a well-stocked and constantly adapting library of virtual resources and vary the activities so it is more than simply a series of documents to read. Ensure your learner knows they are there to be used and guide them towards it whenever appropriate. In doing this we can help our learners find useful and effective ways to meet their learning needs in the virtual world.

Skills, Active Experimentation (AE) 1: PP15

In addition to building up virtual resources there is the more fundamental issue of ensuring that the virtual environment is not obstructive to learning on the job. To a certain extent this is logistical: is the use of the computer system part of the induction process? Or is it left to learners to prise a username and password from the IT department five weeks into the job? Despite what some teenagers may believe, computer access is not a survival need in the physiological sense of food and water. However, in the modern healthcare workplace (and therefore lifelong learning environment), computer access is necessary for survival – it is very difficult for learners if they are constantly 'borrowing' passwords which will discourage from a self-directed approach. Wherever possible learners should be allowed to have control over their own virtual space in the same way they would want control over their

---

Virtual access

Ensure learners are quickly provided with usernames and passwords to their own computer profiles. This allows them control over their virtual learning space, therefore making it a more hassle-free environment. Ensure learners recognise the importance of the virtual world in the modern workplace learning environment.

Motivation, Physiological (P) 2: PP16

physical environment. This means their own profiles with their own desktop, settings and documents. Learners may want to build up a list of 'bookmarks', or access their own browsing history, they could save useful documents and generally set up their profile so that the virtual environment is a comfortable place to be. Without this set-up, learners are likely to continue 'hot-desking' their log-ins and not settling into their own virtual space.

The general ambience

You know the feeling you get in some workplaces or teams – that slightly buzzing feeling that says 'Yes! Go and do it! Is there something new to be learned? Something different to be tried? Let's find it and try it.' This type of atmosphere is in stark contrast to the feel of other workplaces that say something more like 'Hmmm. Do we really have to? Is it absolutely necessary? Why don't we just stick with the status quo? What we are doing is just fine.' More of a 'phut' than a 'buzz'. It is relatively obvious to see that a learner in the latter environment is unlikely to feel they are part of a learning and thriving team and therefore less likely to feel able or willing to develop a self-directed approach. But how on earth can we describe this 'feel' of a place? Most likely you already know whereabouts on the spectrum from 'phut' to 'buzz' your learning environment lies. After all you are part of it. What we are interested in is how this general ambience will impact upon the learner and how it can be used as part of our marginal gains approach to developing their level of self-directedness.

So if we accept that we recognise the feel of a positive learning environment, how can we go about identifying the components that make it up? Especially if we also accept that, like the physical environment (and possibly more so), different people will perceive things differently. We cannot be expected to substantially and fundamentally adapt our workplaces to meet the perceived general ambience needs of each trainee. We could, however, devote some time to discuss the general idea with a few different people and therefore uncover some generalisations about our own specific workplaces. To do this, I would suggest using an adaptation of Personal Construct Theory by Kelly.[29] This tool can be, and is, widely used and complexly analysed, but for our purposes it serves as a method to structure an otherwise vague conversation.

The Repertory Grid

The Repertory Grid is one of the most widely used tools in psychology for instigating discussion and identifying individual constructs. You may recall from Chapter 1, Kelly suggested that we all build constructs to help us analyse the world around us. These constructs are based upon our experiences and they are used to make predictions about future events which may, or may not, result in adaptation of the relevant constructs. So we are going to use the Repertory Grid method to investigate the constructs that people build up around their places of learning (*see* Table 3.4). First identify a number of different learning places, which should include the current space and three or more other learning environments. These could be current, past, at home or any other relevant comparison to the learning environment that the individual has experienced regularly. These form the elements that will make up the headings to the columns in our grid and there should be a minimum of four.

TABLE 3.4 Using a Repertory Grid for analysis of learning environments

Emergent pole of the construct (openly identified in discussion)	Implicit pole of the construct (opposite situation implied by the discussion)	Current workplace	Former workplace 1	Home work space	Alternative working environment

The individual should be given three of the elements (learning spaces) and asked to answer the following question: 'How are two of these alike and different to the third?' The subsequent discussion should identify a similarity between two of the learning spaces (the emergent pole) and by elimination a difference from the third (the implicit pole). Repeat this process with different triads of elements and continue until the individual cannot identify any further similarities or differences. Complete the grid with ticks and crosses for each element and construct. While it is important that the individual comes up with their own constructs as this will demonstrate their priorities, some examples might include:

- willing to try new things (implicit pole: unwilling to try new things)
- take lunch together (implicit pole: lunch eaten in separate rooms)
- team events regularly (implicit pole: few work events)
- encouraged to attend courses (implicit pole: not encouraged to attend courses)
- communal tea/coffee area (implicit pole: people rarely take tea/coffee together)
- lot of others learning (implicit pole: few other people taking part in professional development)
- people at different levels of the organisation learning (implicit pole: only a few higher/middle/lower level staff learning)
- easy to obtain funding for professional development (implicit pole: difficult to obtain funding).

Once the construction of the grid has reached its natural conclusion, you can use this as a starting point to draw out current factors that might contribute to a buzzing learning environment that would encourage self-directedness and what you could learn from other environments experienced by your learners or colleagues. It will also develop the learner's understanding of their own preferences for learning environments. This insight will allow them to identify ways to modify current and future working or learning environments to allow them to develop towards their own chosen goals.

Positive learning atmosphere

Use a Repertory Grid as the structure for a discussion with current and past learners to identify the positive and negative factors in your learning space. Allow your learners to develop insight into their own preferences for the general ambience in a learning space.

Motivation, Self-Actualisation (SA) 3: PP17

Investors in people

Okay, so you don't actually have to get the badge but the general idea of investing in staff has obvious and proven positive impact on businesses. This involves a robust and useful professional development process, open encouragement to learn and to attend courses and, where possible, making funding available for this. It is common sense really: staff who feel they are learning, progressing and being allowed to develop in a direction that is important to them and to their role in the organisation will be more engaged with their workplace. There will be those who do not appear to want to learn, but the chances are, if you can convince them, once they achieve and get a taste for success they will hop on board as well. This idea really belongs in Chapter 7 so we won't dwell on it here except to note that when a learner sees other members of staff learning they are more likely to develop a self-directed approach to their learning. Bandura[30] described how an individual's level of self-efficacy can be raised by seeing others achieving. This increase was maximised when they were observing their direct peers or when they saw many widely differing people succeed. Therefore, observing colleagues and peers of all grades identifying and taking part in learning opportunities will raise a learner's level of self-efficacy.

Learning for all

Develop a learning atmosphere in the team or workplace where all individuals are supported and encouraged to improve and take up learning opportunities. This open demonstration of lifelong learning will help encourage self-directedness in a new learner.

Self-belief, Vicarious Experience (VE) 1: PP18

The three R's

We will make an assumption that our learners have the three Rs (Reading, wRiting and 'Rithmetic) sorted and instead consider the three Rs described by Hiemstra and Sisco.[31] Their three Rs relate to relationships that a learner will develop during their learning experience:

- Relationship with other learners
- Relationship with the instructor
- Relationship with the content of the learning

The combination of these will form a significant part of the general ambience. Perhaps there is more than one learner in your learning environment, team or workplace and if a certain level of camaraderie is fostered this can contribute to a positive feel for the learners. If this is not the case, maybe the current learner could be introduced to former learners and encouraged to keep contact. Either way, learners that have a sense of belonging both within their working team and as part of a learning set can feel secure enough to push forward to learn new things, to take small risks with their learning that will move them onwards and upwards. The same applies to the relationship with their educator – if this is positive and the learner feels supported, they will be more willing to seek out challenge in a self-directed manner. Let's face it, it is much easier to step out and take risks from a safe base; most of us need this to some extent to help us overcome our fear of failure.

Relationships

Encourage learners to develop positive relationships with other learners past or present, within the same team or from other teams. This will help provide the support network the learner needs to have the confidence to identify their own weaknesses and find opportunities to meet the requisite learning needs.

Motivation, Belongingness (B) 2: PP19

The third of our three Rs is the learner's relationship with the content of the learning. We will consider this aspect in much more detail in Chapter 6 where we will look at the importance of involving the learner in the construction of their own curriculum and using feedback on learning from one teaching encounter to inform future teaching.

SUMMARY

So in our brief skim through people and places we have already touched upon research from psychology, management, business, classroom and wider education. We have looked at the learner as a whole person with a multifaceted personality and the learner as a learner with different learning styles and needs. We have also considered three aspects to the learning environment: the physical environment, the virtual environment and the general ambience of a working or learning environment. Throughout all the various considerations that can be used to help develop self-directedness there is one overriding theme: keep the learner in the loop. It is not the intention that educators should rush off and find out their learners VARK[16] preferences, their Honey and Mumford[17] learning style, their Myers-Briggs[7] type, their preferences for physical surroundings, how they perceive different aspects of their workplace and then keep it all in a secret folder on the shelf never to be accessed again. We are trying to develop self-directed learning so everything that we might want to know about our learners as their educator is information they will need to know about themselves. Our learners must develop insight into themselves as learners and this can only be done if we are willing to share what we find in working with them as their teacher and mentor.

In the next chapter we will look more closely at the relationship between the educator and the learner by taking our search for bricks into the realm of mentoring and coaching. The educator–learner relationship will be key to the development of self-directedness and this area of research has plenty of ideas that we can use to help us generate a relationship that encourages a self-directed approach in our learners.

CHAPTER 4

Mentoring and coaching

'It's not differences that divide us. It's our judgements that do. Curiosity and good listening bring us back together.'[1]

INTRODUCTION

It is impossible to consider the medical educator's role in developing self-directedness without looking more closely at the mentoring and coaching strategies that are available to us. Research into mentoring and coaching has really exploded since the 1990s. The idea of 'top-down' learning and management has generally slipped out of favour and in its place mentoring and coaching approaches have taken the fore. There are many and various situations where people will label themselves, or find themselves labelled, with the title of 'mentor' or 'coach'.

The generally accepted forms of the two roles today are the result of many different influences from different realms of research.[2] We will treat the two as separate in this chapter for the sake of simplicity, but in reality there is significant overlap between the roles and the skills involved in both. Fundamentally, both mentoring and coaching are about allowing the learner to maximise their performance. This is achieved by reducing the interfering factors that inhibit their potential: 'Performance = potential − interference'.[3 (p. 17)] There are hundreds of techniques that experienced mentors and coaches will use and we do not have the space to consider them all. However, we will touch upon the key areas of interest to us and look at some suggested tools to help us develop self-directedness in our learners.

MENTORING VS COACHING

As already stated there are significant overlaps between the definitions of mentor and coach and also in the skills required to be an effective mentor or coach. Even a cursory look at the relevant literature reveals a minefield of different definitions. No two are the same and there is significant blurring of the lines between a mentor and a coach. To a certain degree these differences do not matter all that much at a ground level as long as the boundaries of the specific, individual relationship are clear to those involved. However, it is a useful exercise to develop a basic understanding of the two roles to allow a variety of approaches and techniques to be used in different contexts.

There are probably three key and generally accepted differences between mentoring and coaching. The first is that mentoring is usually a 'top-down' affair, and it is most likely that the mentor will be a more senior or at the very least more experienced colleague. The relationship is not and often cannot be an equal partnership because of the nature of the different statuses held within the workplace. The coaching relationship should be an equal partnership where, if anything, the power lies with the coachee because they are seen to hold the solutions for themselves (for reasons that I cannot explain I find the word 'coachee' unsatisfying but there is no other sensible alternative so let's run with it). While a mentee (that's not much better, it sounds like a mint-flavoured sweet) might bring a problem to their mentor and be provided with a solution or a means to find the solution, a coachee would be questioned until they uncover the solution or means to find it for themselves.

The second key difference between mentoring and coaching relationships is the length of time over which the relationship takes place. A mentoring relationship is generally a long-term relationship, therefore many of these bricks relate to longer term training or induction processes rather than brief learning encounters. Coaching skills, however, can be used in a much shorter relationship; in fact there are even some techniques that could be used in a one-off encounter.

Third, another important distinction is in the level of craft knowledge: a mentor will be an individual with specific knowledge of the job; they will have a high level of relevant expertise which they can convey to their mentee in a number of different ways. Of course knowing the answer does not have to mean handing it over in a manner that encourages dependent learners and obstructs the development of self-directedness. The coach, meanwhile, does not need (and is arguably better off without) this type of knowledge. At the core of coaching is the belief that the coachee holds the necessary knowledge to solve their problem. If the learner does not have the exact knowledge required they should be able to work out where to find it and therefore uncover their own solutions.

> A mentor is usually an expert in a particular field and works with more junior practitioners in that field, helping them to gain knowledge, skills and experience.
>   Coaching is about facilitating self-directed learning and development. The coach does not necessarily have specific expertise in the area of influence of the

person he or she is coaching. Sometimes not having expertise in the working area of a client allows valuable insight.[4 (p. 16)]

Of course life is not even this simple, as there are many (many) different types of learning relationship and they can rarely be so cleanly categorised into 'mentor' or 'coach' especially in the sometimes frantic working environment. Table 4.1, produced by Bayley,[5] demonstrates some of this variety and the areas of overlap between roles.

TABLE 4.1 A comparison of the roles and requirements of different learning relationships

Role	Characteristics of role and responsibilities						
	One to one	Group	Long term	Short term	Management led	Personal development	Professional development
Coach	X			X		X	X
Mentor	X		X			X	X
Preceptor	X			X			X
Assessor	X			X	X		X
Clinical Supervisor	X	X	X			X	X
Appraiser	X			X	X		X

To make things additionally complicated, it is common in medical education for an individual to find themselves taking on more than one of these roles within a single learning relationship. Clinical supervisors are often assessors and it is unlikely that any of these roles are without at least a touch of mentorship. So what can we actually take away from these attempts to lay down the borders between roles? We get a clearer picture of the type of relationship we are building and when it is appropriate to take on these different roles in a more clearly defined manner. Defining the sort of relationship you are working towards helps both you and the learner settle more easily into compatible roles within the relationship.

NEEDS ANALYSIS

Before we begin looking in detail at the two roles we should keep in mind the general environment within which we are mentoring or coaching: in particular the 'needs' environment. Tulpa put together a diagram to emphasise the importance of the alignment of needs when taking part in organisational coaching. Figure 4.1 shows an adaptation of this idea for the realm of medical education.[6]

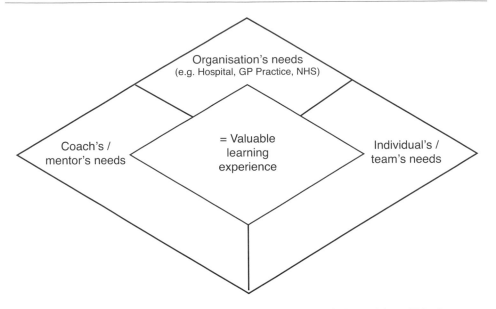

FIGURE 4.1 The needs environment for medical education (adapted from Tulpa)

One of the potential issues with self-directedness identified in Chapter 2 was self-directedness to the detriment of the team. It is clearly easiest to motivate an individual towards their own personal gain; however, it will be more difficult to achieve if the individual's identified needs are in opposition to those of the team and/or the organisation. Discussion of the wider context at a suitable point in a learning conversation will help bring together the needs of all concerned. Ideally everyone will be pulling in the same direction and the learner will identify learning needs based upon their own interests or areas of weakness that match with the needs of the team and organisation in which they work. These needs will tie in with the mentor or coach's development profile: either existing within the mentor's area of expertise or requiring skills that the mentor or coach is willing and able to develop. With this level of 'needs' congruence, the learner will be able to move forward supported by the wider context. If there is little or no overlap the learner will at best have to work very independently and at worst they may find barriers placed in their path.

Congruent objectives

Ensure that the individual identified learning needs are not in direct opposition to those of the team, coach/mentor or organisation. This will help ensure the success of the learner when they attempt a learning task by increasing the level and breadth of support they receive.

Self-belief, Performance Accomplishments (PA) 2: MC1

MENTORING

The term 'mentor' and the associated role has become very significant in healthcare. It is often used in the formal learning environment; for example, nurses and mid-wives are assigned specific 'mentors' during their training. In addition to being a role for experienced staff to guide new staff, many of the organisations involved in medical education (Royal Colleges, government organisations, academic organisa-tions) have set up their own mentoring programmes. The reasoning behind such a wide take-up of mentoring is made clear by Bayley et al.[5]

> Fostering a mentoring relationship develops, supports and equips staff with the skills they need to:
> - support changes and improvements in patient care
> - take advantage of wider care opportunities
> - realise their potential.[5 (p. 6)]

Defining the role of the mentor

To fully understand the role of mentoring in developing self-directedness we need to describe a mentor, and there are enough definitions out there to fill an entire book. However, if I did that your eyeballs would probably melt out of their sockets in boredom. Instead we will take a brief look at a handful of descriptions to give a taste of the variety out there. First up, Anderson and Shannon[7] identify a number of aspects of a mentor:

- nurturing (appropriate support for growth, considering the personality as a whole)
- ongoing caring relationship (like a parent–child relationship)
- basic mentoring functions (teacher, sponsor, encourager, counsellor, befriender)
- focus on professional and personal development (concern regarding trainee welfare)
- role modelling (development by example).

Watkins[8] described the knowledge required of a teaching mentor and this can be usefully adapted for medical educators. These five areas of knowledge primarily relate to the initial training or induction context, but they also have a secondary role in the mentoring of more experienced individuals.

- A mentor must have an understanding of the role of the clinician: dissection of understanding of their own knowledge, skills and role, in order to role model the job.
- A mentor must have an understanding of how learners learn about the patient encounter: knowledge of the reflective process and role modelling reflection.
- A mentor must have an understanding of the non-patient aspects of the clinician's

role: being a clinician of any sort involves significantly more than the patient encounters. There is always the paperwork. And the meetings. And the paperwork. And the politics. And of course the paperwork. It is important that learners are aware of the level of administrative work and the wide variety of liaison with colleagues that is also involved. Otherwise there is a risk that they will complete their training with a narrow view of the role.

- A mentor must have an understanding of the concerns and experiences of new trainees: as well as concerns over subject knowledge and managing patients, trainees are often concerned about how they will fit into their new environment. They are expected to assimilate a lot of information in a short period of time when they begin a placement which can be challenging.

- A mentor must have an understanding of how one adult may help another learn (the task dimension and the skills dimension):
  - ○ The task dimension is the training programme that the mentor puts into place. This could include observations both by and of the learner, and discussion of patient encounters in which reflective practice is encouraged. Focused observations tend to be more useful for a trainee as they help them work towards specific targets. Discussion of the learning process is also very important because both mentors and trainees should be able to describe how well learning outcomes have been met and what the future learning needs are.
  - ○ The skills dimension is those skills required to be a successful mentor; to set up a supportive environment where good communication, specific and challenging targets and constructive feedback lead to development of the trainee.

Formal vs informal mentoring

Mentoring is so much part of the modern day healthcare education process that there is a significant chance that you have already been a mentor or a mentee. There is also a possibility that you may not have even been aware of this process. It is not uncommon for people to gravitate towards someone who is more experienced and who is willing to spend a little time guiding a less experienced colleague. Golian and Galbraith[9] describe the two forms that mentoring can take: formal and informal.

> Informal mentoring is a relationship that occurs that is unplanned, and, in most cases, not expected. A certain 'chemistry' emerges drawing two individuals together for the purpose of professional, personal and psychological growth and development. Informal mentoring seems to be a qualitative experience that has great meaning for the parties involved.[9 (p. 10)]

By contrast, formal or sponsored mentoring 'is a method designed to reach a variety of specific goals and purposes, defined within the setting in which it operates.'[9 (p. 10)]

Table 4.2[10] gives a very practical definition of what mentors do but also provides a reflective opportunity. Look at formal mentoring relationships that you have been part of and identify times when you may have been mentored informally.

TABLE 4.2 A tool for reflection on your role in mentor–mentee relationships

Mentors ...	Others have done this for me	I have done this for others
Set high performance expectations		
Offer challenging ideas		
Help build self-confidence		
Encourage professional behaviour		
Offer friendship		
Confront negative behaviours and attitudes		
Listen to personal problems		
Teach by example		
Provide growth experiences		
Offer quotable quotes		
Explain how the organisation works		
Help far beyond their duties or obligations		
Stand by their mentees in critical situations		
Offer wise counsel		
Encourage winning behaviour		
Trigger self-awareness		
Inspire to excellence		
Share critical knowledge		
Offer encouragement		
Assist with careers		

Awareness of mentoring

Discuss with your learner times when they have been in a mentoring relationship and dissect what was involved and what worked (or didn't). An awareness of this type of role may encourage them to seek out mentoring-style relationships throughout their career so providing opportunities for additional support in the road to self-directedness.

Self-belief, Verbal Persuasion (VP) 3: MC2

The last (I promise) look at the role of the mentor comes from Cohen,[11] who identifies six ingredients for the mentor as described in Table 4.3.

TABLE 4.3 Six functions of a mentor according to Cohen[11]

Function	Description of the function/skills used by the mentor	How this contributes to the development of self-directedness
Relationship emphasis	The mentor uses active listening skills and an empathetic approach to develop an understanding of the mentee's emotional state. Open questions and a non-judgemental approach help to generate an open relationship that is based on a trusting and reflective process. The mentor is responsive to the mentee and their worries.	By building an honest, open and trusting relationship the learner feels safe enough to take risks with their learning in a way that will be necessary for self-directed learning.
Information emphasis	The mentor will ask for detailed information and may provide information in the form of advice as part of this function. The mentor may use closed questions in a clear fact-gathering exercise.	This type of discussion demonstrates to learners the many different factors they need to consider when defining their own learning needs. It models the probing questions they need to ask themselves (i.e. the reflective processes) in order to clearly define a problem or concern.
Facilitative focus	This function expands on the factual collection to encourage the mentee to review their own interests and beliefs. The aim is to encourage more creativity in considering alternative learning objectives and how these might be achieved. The mentor promotes a very reflective approach through hypothetical questioning.	Within this function the mentor is developing the creativity of the learner in terms of finding alternative means to meet their chosen endpoint. The mentor helps the mentee to place their new understanding within a different context or construct that expands the mentee's view.
Confrontative focus	The mentor must first carefully consider the learner's readiness for challenge. The mentor challenges decisions, explanations or actions (or lack thereof) made by the mentee. This focus encourages critical thinking and discussion in a respectful environment.	This focus further develops a reflective, insightful process in learners by encouraging deep, critical thought about their own reasoning and justifications for decisions and actions.

Function	Description of the function/skills used by the mentor	How this contributes to the development of self-directedness
Modelling	The mentor shares their own experiences and those of other mentees to demonstrate both past successes and learning from past mistakes. The mentor provides realistic assessments of the learner's abilities and encourages appropriate risk taking with learning.	Through modelling in this way the mentor provides vicarious experiences that will help increase the learner's level of self-efficacy. Especially if the experiences of other mentees are used whom the learner may see as a peer.
Visioning	The mentor steers conversations towards envisioning the future in a critical manner. The mentor makes statements that require the mentee to reflect on future education, training and career. There is consideration of the potential impact of actions on personal and professional life. Questioning elicits understanding of the different hypothetical outcomes and perspectives (positive and negative). The mentor is always respectful of the mentee's final decision and their ability to make these decisions.	Through this process the learner develops their ability to critically consider the multitude of options available. Being led through by a mentor enables them to develop the skills to navigate this process themselves in future learning. The respect shown to the mentee's decisions develops their sense of autonomy and their level of self-efficacy.

There are many different things to take from this dissection of the mentoring role, a number of which will nurture a self-directed approach by our learners.

The mentor–mentee relationship

Build an open and honest relationship by making the relationship itself a key focus of the mentor role. Active listening, empathy, open questions and a non-judgemental approach will all help build a trusting relationship in which the learner feels secure.

Motivation, Safety (S) 3: MC3

The modelling mentor

When acting as a mentor, role model possible approaches and outcomes; this can be done either through your own actions or those of other learners. Demonstrate a willingness to learn from mistakes and from the mistakes of others.

Self-belief, Vicarious Experience (VE) 2: MC4

A critical visioning approach

When discussing learning with the learner challenge them to think about hypothetical situations and the potential impacts of different approaches. Encourage
them, through questioning, to critique their decisions from all perspectives.

Skills, Abstract Conceptualisation (AC) 2: MC5

Stages of mentoring

Okay. So I maybe fudged that last promise a little; we will take a quick look at the
process of mentoring. Instead of looking at the specific definition of the role, we will
be looking at how the role develops as time progresses. So, technically, the Cohen/
Galbraith discussion was the last bit on defining the role of the mentor. Really.
Honestly.

When we look at coaching conversations there will be a significant amount of text
given to the details of the actual coaching conversation. In coaching there is a lot of
consideration given to the overall conversational structure, the style of questions and
the language used. It therefore seems only fair to give a brief recognition to the structure of the mentoring process; Parsloe and Leedham[2] suggest a four-stage process:

1. Analysing for awareness of need, desire and self.
2. Planning for self-responsibility.
3. Implementing using styles, techniques and skills.
4. Evaluating for success and learning.[2 (p. 21)]

This overall description of the stages of mentoring provides a useful basic structure
on which we can place our learning conversations. As we shall see it also bears a
marked resemblance to the overall structure of coaching processes.

COACHING

Although much of the modern mentoring literature describes a good mentor as being
one that asks probing questions to elicit information from the mentee, this actually
demonstrates a slide towards a coaching approach. The traditional use of the term
'mentor' – the advice-giving expert – exists at the opposite end of a continuum to a
coach. In a coaching conversation the coach provides the process while the coachee
provides the actual content. This is in contrast to the far end of the continuum in
'traditional mentoring' where the content will, at least in part, come from the mentor.

Alexander[12] identifies three areas of competence for coaches: relationship, being and doing. First, in order to build a positive relationship, the coach must be open and honest as discussed in the relationship emphasis of Cohen's[11] mentoring functions. The second area relates to the coach's state of mind and their level of self-confidence. They must believe they are able to support the trainee through difficulties and have the self-awareness and insight into their own abilities and approaches. Finally the 'doing' competencies are those tools and techniques that a coach might use in a coaching conversation. It is on these final competencies that we will mostly focus the rest of this section as this is where we find the practical advice to help develop self-directedness. However, it is important to recognise that coaches themselves must feel confident that they are able to meet the learner needs. If after reflection an educator feels they may be out of their depth in general or with a specific learner, they should consider asking for an education mentor. This will be someone with the experience and necessary skills to support the educator in supporting the learner. If the educator lacks self-confidence it is likely that the learner will not feel confident in their educator and may feel insecure in their learning.

A confident educator

Learners will benefit from an educator who is confident in their ability to provide support. This does not mean knowing all the answers; instead they should be content to admit they do not know the answer and make it clear this is not a failure. The learner can feel confident in their educator and trust in their ability and their openness.

Self-belief, Verbal Persuasion (VP) 4: MC6

Establishing rapport

> Rapport is like money: it increases in importance when you do not have it, and when you do have it, a lot of opportunities appear.[13 (p. 27)]

First, within Alexander's[12] 'relationship' competence for coaches, we will look at rapport. Building rapport is key for the development of an open and trusting relationship that is the basis for effective learning conversations. It is unfortunately a very intangible thing. I have seen plenty of learning relationships break down, and occasionally this is the result of a specific incident, but more often it is down to a lack of 'fit' between the educator and the learner. It is something that no one can really put their finger on and is often put down to a 'personality clash'. In actuality it is often due to poor rapport building, as the learner and the educator feel the differences between them rather than the similarities.

Laborde[13] proposes a number of levels of rapport – it is a useful reflective point to consider where on this scale your learning relationships lie:

- Seduction(!)
- Hot
- Cosily warm
- **Warm**
- **Identification**
- **Understanding**
- **Lukewarm**
- **Neutral**
- Cool
- Sufferance

On this scale neutral to warm is the region that is best for business. There are two inextricably linked and easily definable reasons for a relationship that exists below neutral: your belief in the learner's ability and the learner's trust in your ability. An educator who does not believe in the competence of the learner is likely to cause increasing resentment. An important part of developing rapport is to ensure that educators demonstrate faith in the ability and the potential of their learners.

Faith in the learner's ability

Ensure strong foundations for a relationship with good rapport by demonstrating a belief in your learner. This is a belief in their ability to obtain the knowledge and skills needed; to achieve the learning objectives and to gain the necessary insight to determine their own learning needs and act towards them. Find a way to provide compliments, whether about the outcome or the process.

Motivation, Self-Esteem (SE) 2: MC7

It is also possible that a lack of rapport is due to a lack of trust in your ability as an educator. If this is the case it is necessary to find a way to establish credibility. Once the learner has come to trust that you are capable of helping them towards their chosen objective you can set about establishing a rapport somewhere between neutral and warm. If you sense that there is a lack of rapport due to a lack of trust, enhance your credibility by sharing your successes with your learner (without appearing to be a total show-off obviously).

Laborde[13] goes on to define a number of areas, which many of us will do instinctively to establish rapport but that we can choose to work on if necessary.

- Matching speech patterns: the tempo and tone can both be taken into account when shifting your speech pattern to be more similar to the learner.
- Matching breathing rates.
- Matching movement rhythms: also known as crossover mirroring, this involves finding your learner's repetitive movement, their 'tell', and then choosing a specific movement that you do each time they make their movement. So if they tuck their hair behind their ear you might stroke your chin.
- Matching body postures.

Now clearly this all needs to be done very subtly or your learner will find themselves faced with an extremely disturbing learning encounter that may scare them enough to avoid ever being alone in a room with you again.

Developing rapport

Develop rapport by subtly matching speech patterns, breathing rates, movement rhythms (crossover mirroring) and body postures. Establishing positive educator–learner relationships now will increase the likelihood of the learner seeking out similar supportive relationships in the future.

Motivation, Belongingness (B) 3: MC8

Developing clear goals

Goal setting fundamentally underpins a coaching conversation and many other learning experiences. There needs to be an explicit reason why you are having the conversation to ensure that both the coach and the coachee are pulling in the same direction. Not all conversations will need a formalised goal-setting approach; however, when sitting down to discuss learning targets or particular problems or concerns of the learner it is important to have a focus to the discussion. Learners will often be quite vague about what they are hoping to gain from the conversation so we need to help them drill down into what they want to achieve. Goals are important for a number of reasons; Locke and Latham[14] described four functions for goals:

1. a directive function – focusing actions in a particular direction
2. an energising function – increased level of effort
3. a persistence function – increased length of time of effort
4. a knowledge function – if the learner already has the skills they will quickly

adapt and use their current knowledge or skills; alternatively a goal allows them to focus their thoughts onto what new knowledge or skills they need to acquire.

Locke and Latham[14] identified a number of patterns to goal-setting research. First there is a directly proportional relationship between the level of difficulty of the target and the levels of effort and performance. There appears to be some conflict at the highest level of this relationship. Some research indicates that at the highest level of difficulty effort and performance drop off because the individual is over-challenged, while others suggest that the positive correlation continues until the goal is actually impossible for the learner to achieve. Second, a key aspect of the goal is specificity, as people achieve most highly when they are provided with specific and challenging goals. Third, Locke described the importance of considering the self-setting of goals in the context of the learner's level of self-efficacy. While there is conflicting research regarding the impact of learner participation in goal setting, learners with a high level of self-efficacy will set more difficult targets.

One of the most widely referenced target writing tools is 'SMART' targeting. The origins of this acronym are unclear, plus I've no doubt that you, like me, have come across more than one alternative of the model. The one presented here is probably the most useful for the medical education context.

S   Specific: make sure that the target is very clear and focused because this will lead to higher performances; avoid vague statements like 'become more experienced'.

M   Measureable: it will be clear when the target has been achieved.

A   Attainable: as previously discussed the goal should be challenging but achievable for the learner.

R   Relevant: it may be relevant to the learner's personal ambitions, professional ambitions, the team or workplace requirements or other mandatory aspects like curriculum demands.

T   Time related: there should be a deadline of some sort for achievement of the goal.

SMART targets

Ensure that targets set for learning are SMART so that learners are clear about what they are aiming for and that they will know when they have achieved it. A specific goal is important for the learner to feel a sense of achievement when they succeed.

Self-belief, Performance Accomplishments (PA) 3: MC9

The coaching conversation structure

There are many different paths to take in a coaching conversation, but one of the most widely used and easily applied is the GROW model. This model was developed by Alexander and Renshaw[12] as a result of reflection on actual coaching sessions. It divides the coaching conversation into four sections that (despite the implication of the acronym) do not have to necessarily be tackled in a linear manner.

- Goal: define a measurable outcome of the session or, if it is a longer relationship, for a longer but defined period of time. This should involve really drilling down into the coachee's specific aims, which may be rather vague at the outset.
- Reality: discuss the situation within which the problem and/or the goal are set. Consider all the variables and perspectives that are impacting upon the problem or on potential solutions.
- Options: it is likely that the discussion of the reality will begin to throw up some options for how to move forwards. Make sure these options are expanded as much as possible then drawn together in a coherent manner.
- Way forward: now the coachee must be encouraged to select one particular action. Through questioning, the coachee should devise a clear plan of attack that they can take away with them and act upon. At this stage it may be supportive to use challenging questions: 'What about …?', 'Have you considered how … will react?', 'What will you do if …?' This helps to ensure that the coachee has thought through their action plan in a critical manner and therefore improve the chances of a positive outcome.

Of course it is not necessary to strictly adhere to the given order; in fact successful coaching conversations are often much less prescribed. A more general approach is what I am going to call the coaching conversation cones (*see* Figure 4.2). The conversation begins relatively open as the general aim of the conversation is narrowed down to a goal that provides the first 'cone'. After this goal-setting process sits the second 'cone'; this is narrow at first then the conversation broadens out in the fluid exploration stage. The widest point of the conversation should be when the potential options are considered then this narrows (the third 'cone') as the potential outcomes are evaluated and some options discarded. Finally the conversation is narrowed to a single action that will initiate the rest of the action plan to make the desired change come about.

This approach can be used by coaches and learners to evaluate learning conversations and develop insight into thinking processes. Perhaps learners do not adequately narrow the conversation at the start or maybe they are not broad enough in their consideration of possible options. It can be easy to dismiss some options because of an unchangeable external factor, but occasionally discussion of even these apparently impossible options leads to a useful adaptation of the context or

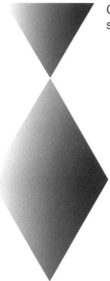

Goal setting for the conversation, narrow down to single goal to achieve in the coaching conversation

Broaden the conversation to explore the situation, different ideas, perspectives, potential solutions

Narrow the conversation down again through the production of a specific action plan

FIGURE 4.2 Coaching conversation cones

the option itself to make it workable. Another common stumbling block is a lack of specificity in action planning; learners need to determine their exact next step to get themselves on the right path.

Insight into their own tendencies within a coaching conversation will help the learner effectively use their time in the car or before they go to bed or walking the dog to work through this process in their own heads. This develops their ability to produce a valid and achievable action plan, one that they can and will carry out within the self-determined time constraints.

Coaching conversation cones

Begin learning conversations with a narrowing process to clearly define the goal of the conversation. Then broaden the conversation again as different perspectives and alternative solutions are discussed. Finally, narrow the conversation right back down again to form a specific plan of action. Give the learner insight into this process to help them develop the skills to action plan for themselves.

Skills, Active Experimentation (AE) 2: MC10

Alexander[15] also suggests some tools for use when coaching conversations are grounded on a particular issue. The 'structure of a problem' exercise is an analytical tool for an empowering discussion of a problem (*see* Figure 4.3).

1. Use post-it notes or index cards to set up a diagram similar to the one in Figure 4.3 through discussion.
2. Encourage the coachee to describe in detail the current state and the desired state, use questions to elicit how these states would appear from different perspectives.
3. Through further questioning get the trainee to identify the barriers to the change from the current state to the desired state. For each barrier they should discuss whether the locus of the barrier is within themselves, with others (identify who exactly) or part of the environment.
4. From this point the discussion can move towards dismantling these barriers. Ideally, the coachee will provide the solutions themselves now that they have a greater understanding of the sources of the obstacles.

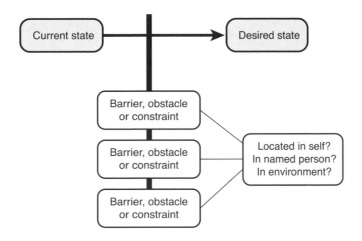

FIGURE 4.3 Structuring the problem (as described by Alexander)

Structuring the problem

Encourage learners to describe their current situation and the desired situation, then discuss the barriers to the change. For each barrier consider whether the locus is within the learner, within another specific individual or part of the environment. This will help develop the learner's thinking skills and provide them with a tool that a learner could use for problem solving on their own.

Skills, Active Experimentation (AE) 3: MC11

Alexander also suggests the use of 'areas of life cards' (*see* Figure 4.4). These are nine cards each containing an area of the coachee's life: family, health, leisure, career, vision, network, finance, development and performance. These are each discussed in turn from three different perspectives: self, observer and a named other.

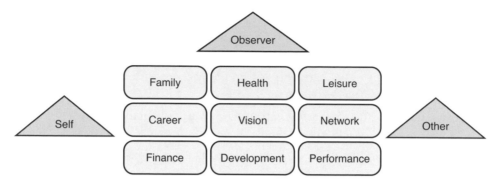

FIGURE 4.4 Areas of life perspectives exercise (as described by Alexander)

Perspectives on life

Each time the learner encounters a problem or a new situation or piece of information, encourage them to think about different aspects of their life (family, health, leisure, career, vision, network, finance, development and performance) from different perspectives (self, unbiased observer plus another named individual).

Skills, Reflective Observation (RO) 3: MC 12

Listening

Good listening is a key skill in any effective relationship which probably explains why 'good listener' is found in so many lonely hearts columns (I mean online dating profiles – showing my age there). There are plenty of people who have tried to develop various 'levels of listening' to help educators and coaches develop a deeper understanding of exactly what it means to be a 'good listener'. Being a good listener cannot be achieved through a checklist of behaviours; however, these models demonstrate the general principles of research into listening behaviours. Although behaviourist researchers may get a little cross with me for distilling a huge area of work into a few quick and dirty descriptions of models, in the space we've got I'm afraid this is probably the most sensible way forward. Sorry.

Research into listening is long standing and in the 1940s the 'ten commandments' of listening were developed based upon identification of the most common features of poor listening.[16]

Thou shalt not:

1. condemn a speaker's subject as uninteresting
2. criticise the speaker's delivery rather than focus on the message
3. prepare an answer to a point or question before comprehending it
4. listen only for facts
5. waste the advantage of thought speed over speech speed
6. tolerate or create distractions
7. fake attention
8. permit personal prejudices to interfere
9. avoid difficult material
10. attempt to take outline notes even when the message isn't structured.

Bresser and Wilson[17] describe five levels of listening (*see* Table 4.4), which are a fair representation of the many possible levels of listening model out there.

TABLE 4.4 Levels of listening

Level 1	Planning what to say instead of listening to what the speaker is saying. This is the most irritating level of listening because the speaker can tell that the listener is not listening.
Level 2	Giving a reply that is about the listener not the speaker. This is probably how the majority of conventional conversations are conducted.
Level 3	Giving advice. This is still more about the listener than the speaker, and can be close to level 1 in the irritation stakes if the speaker is looking for a sympathetic ear rather than direction.
Level 4	Listening and inviting more. People often work things out while they are talking and a prompt from the coach may help the flow.
Level 5	Listening behind and between the words; listening to the silences; using one's intuition.[17 (p. 17)]

These two approaches to describing good listening identify some of the common pitfalls of listening that we are probably all guilty of at one time or another. Hands up if you have caught yourself thinking about what you are going to say instead of actually listening; giving replies that draw the conversation back to you; giving advice inappropriately? I'm guilty of it sometimes. One of the key aspects of coaching for self-directedness is that the learner needs to be guided towards developing their own solutions. This way they will improve their ability to problem solve, plus when it is their own solution they are more likely to attempt it with the level of commitment required for success.

Another interesting model of listening is the HURIER model by Brownell.[18] This is not another 'levels of listening' model, instead it describes the process of effective listening: Hearing, Understanding, Remembering, Interpreting, Evaluating and

Responding. It is interesting to note that the response is the very last thing on this list, as the final reply by the listener is based upon information gathered through the previous five stages of listening. It is very easy to get caught up in thinking about how to respond and in doing so skip the understanding, remembering, interpreting, evaluating stages.

- Hearing: the physical process of hearing. Are you able to focus on the information you should be listening to? Or do you find yourself easily distracted by other noises or starting to glaze over so the information goes in one ear and out the other?

- Understanding: the message has been received but how well did you understand it on a literal level? At this point language and literacy and even cultural references can be a barrier to listening.

- Remembering: depending on your preferred learning style you may find it difficult to take on board information that is presented orally in this manner (I know I do). How well could you recap the information you have just received? You can only respond using the information that you can recall.

- Interpreting: the interpretation of both verbal and non-verbal cues. How well do you take note of facial expressions, tone of voice, body language? This must also be placed into the wider context.

- Evaluating: this final stage before the response requires the listener to pull together all the information and form a judgement; it is key that this judgement only happens after the collection of all information.

- Responding: the response will be whatever the listener now deems appropriate; it is important to remember that the response will be both verbal and non-verbal and that the listener should continue to listen (particularly to non-verbal cues) while they are responding, thus giving a process of continual listening.

Active listening

Listen actively to your learner and in doing so encourage them to be forthcoming with their thoughts and feelings. By listening in a positive manner the learner is made to feel that their thoughts are valuable.

Motivation, Self-Esteem (SE) 3: MC13

Asking good questions

Most of us are familiar with the idea of open and closed questions. An open question allows the learner to give many possible answers that could direct the conversation in any direction. These questions will need more than a one word answer. Using open questions in learning conversations allows the learner to develop the skills to negotiate their own learning. However, thinking of these questions in the middle of a conversation is often not as easy as it should be. Whitmore[19] produced a series of generic and simple questions that could be used to further a conversation.

- 'What else?'
- 'If you knew the answer what would it be?'
- 'What would the consequences of that be for you or for others?'
- 'What criteria are you using?'
- 'What is the hardest/most challenging part of this for you?'
- 'What advice would you give a friend in this situation?'
- 'Imagine having a dialogue with the wisest person you know or can think of. What would he or she tell you to do?'
- 'I don't know where to go next with this. Where would you go?'
- 'What would you gain/lose by doing/saying that?'
- 'If someone said/did that to you, what would you feel/think/do?'[19 (pp. 51–2)]

Powerful questioning is an absolute must for the development of self-directedness. Without good questioning the conversation quickly becomes advice giving, which is not conducive for self-directedness. Questioning is a skill that needs to be developed and improved in the same way as any other skill. There is plenty of material out there to draw on but, ultimately, practice and reflection are the most useful tools. Many pieces of literature will point to the 'magic' question, finding the one question that unlocks the whole issue. Sometimes there is a magic turning point in the conversation, but often there will be many dead ends before the depth of the problem is fully appreciated and a successful solution and action plan is settled upon. That is why the art of questioning is so important for developing self-directedness; the learner has to be allowed to work out by trial and error the variety of options available to them. For each one they need to determine the likelihood of success by evaluating potential outcomes.

Open questioning

Use high-quality open questioning to develop the learner's thinking skills. Questions should encourage thinking from multiple perspectives, both time and person. Give learners the space to expand their thoughts in a way that encourages them to develop their thinking skills.

Skills, Abstract Conceptualisation (AC) 3: MC14

Types of coaching

There are many, many different types of coaching that each describe a slightly different set of principles. However, once you get down to ground level the differences diminish. Each of them will use the skills already discussed: rapport building, goal setting, questioning and in reality each type of coaching is a useful string on the proverbial bow.

Solution-focused coaching

The standard style of coaching conversation will usually involve spending a significant amount of time analysing the problem whereas in solution-focused coaching this idea is turned on its head. Once the problem has been identified the conversation is switched to other contexts where the problem does not manifest itself. The aim is to identify attributes and skills that the learner has demonstrated in alternative contexts then work out how to transfer them to create a solution in the problematical context.

> This is why the solution-focused approach is so important. Focusing on solutions means that you use the solutions that are happening *anyway* and build on these. ... By dwelling on the causes of problems we often perpetuate and exaggerate them. Over-engaging in self-reflection and focusing on problems actually makes us feel worse. By looking for solutions we immediately shift the emphasis from the past to the future.[4 (p. 28)]

This is a particularly positive approach to coaching and is one that learners may find useful in trying to problem solve for themselves. It teaches them to hunt through the different contexts in their lives for solutions that use skills they already have.

A solution-focused approach

Demonstrate a solution-focused approach to problem solving to allow learners to develop the skill of looking at their current skill set to find a solution. Encourage them to look at different contexts within their life to find somewhere that the problem does not manifest itself.

Skills, Active Experimentation (AE) 4: MC15

Cognitive coaching

Cognitive coaching is a fascinating approach to coaching devised by Costa and Garmston[20] based upon the concept of holonomy – the wholeness of people. The cognitive coach attempts to develop the five identified states of mind: efficacy, flex-ibility, consciousness, craftsmanship and interdependence. At the heart of this approach are a number of tensions that exist within all people as they attempt to balance the art of being independent individuals expressing their own uniqueness while living within constraining systems that permit and restrict certain behaviours. This is described as independence vs community.[21] There are a number of tensions that arise as a result of this balancing act that are an interesting background to our work with learners:

- ambiguity vs certainty
- knowledge vs action
- egocentricity vs allocentricity
- self-assertion vs integration
- inner feelings vs outer behaviours
- solitude vs interconnectedness

When learners find themselves caught between the proverbial rock and a hard place they will likely find themselves stressed and anxious about their decision making. A cognitive coach aims to help the coachee manage this balancing act and in doing so create an individual capable of controlling their anxieties.

Individuality vs community

Learners (like everyone) are caught in a tension between their drive to be inde-pendent individuals and the constraints of being a member of many wider communities. Help learners develop insights into their greatest challenges in this balancing act and develop strategies to deal with the fine line they are treading.

Self-belief, Emotional Arousal (EA) 3: MC16

Cognitive coaching is all about mental processes occurring within the individual's mind and whether these are self-enhancing or self-defeating. There are a number of specific thought processes, called negative automatic thoughts, which we should be aware of as they are particularly self-defeating.

- All or nothing thinking: 'Pass or fail', 'win or lose'
- Mind reading: making assumptions about other people's thoughts based upon incomplete information
- Fortune telling: 'I know it will be awful'
- Magnification/catastrophising: 'The world is ending'
- Personalisation: 'This is all about me/my actions'

- Negative feedback loops: feeling 'Thank goodness that's over' instead of feeling energised by an achievement
- Discounting the positive: 'If I can do it, it doesn't count'
- Laying blame: with themselves or with others
- Generalisations: 'I never get what I want', 'It's always the same'.

These thought processes can be challenged using a combination of evidence, logic and pragmatism. Bringing the learner's attention to these processes will not only help them in the immediate task but also in self-identification of these thoughts in the future.

Negative automatic thoughts

Challenge negative thought processes in your learner using logic, evidence and pragmatism. Encourage them to recognise these self-defeating thoughts in themselves and learn how to correct them in real time to promote positive reflection-in-action.

Skills, Reflective Observation (RO) 4: MC17

Transactional analysis

Berne's[22] Parent, Adult, Child ego states model provides another approach to coaching conversations. We first looked at this theory to help us understand our learner's individual psyche, but it is usually applied to conversations in the form of transactional analysis. The term transactional analysis is a result of Berne's analysis of conversations as transactions. He described conversations as a process in which the speakers unconsciously decide upon a level of detail expected by both sides then a transaction takes place with an appropriate level of information. If one side provides more or less information than the other expects the result is surprise: 'What is wrong with him today?!' for one reason or another.

Straightforward conversations are adult to adult (type 1) and parent to child (type 2) – these transactions are complementary and follow a natural order so they should proceed smoothly and indefinitely. It is instinctive that the adult–adult conversations are the most useful for developing self-directedness. When crossed transactions occur communication will likely be broken off as the ego states involved are incompatible and until one of the people involved shifts their ego state it will probably be rather uncomfortable.

This analysis becomes more complex when there are ulterior transactions. In these conversations there are more than two ego states involved. Although the conversation may appear to be progressing on an adult–adult level there are actually other ego states involved. For example:

> 'I wonder how we can improve the experience of children in the hospital waiting room.'
>
> 'Well I remember playing with an etch-a-sketch at hospital when I broke my leg as a child.'
>
> 'I remember etch-a-sketches; I used to love mine! We could look at asking for donations.'

This is an adult to adult conversation, but it is also communicating at the child level because of the memories involved.

Transactional analysis is a handy tool for dissection of our learning conversations. If we approach a conversation as a parent we may encourage the child ego state in our learners, which is counter-productive in developing self-directedness. Equally, if a learner appears to be in their child state, responding as a parent will encourage the 'child' to either adapt to the feedback without deeper thinking or to rebel against the feedback. We should aim for conversations between adult ego states that allow rational, reflective discussions to take place that result in structured and progressive learning targets. If a learner is in their adult state of mind throughout a learning conversation they are more likely to produce an achievable action plan that they actively pursue.

Transactional analysis

Use Berne's ego states to analyse learning conversations. This will help you as the educator to have effective and complementary conversations with the learner. The learner should be encouraged to be in their adult state to set their own targets and produce the action plan to improve the chances of success.

Self-Belief: Performance Accomplishments (PA) 4: MC18

Sports coaching

It would be wrong to finish a section on coaching without mentioning the root of coaching: sports coaching. Things have moved on from the scary bloke with a whistle barking 'Another lap' on the coldest day of the year while you wear ridiculously small gym knickers. Sports psychology is a huge area of research, but we will draw on just one particularly useful approach for our model of self-directedness.

Visualisation gets rugby balls through the posts in World Cup matches, it puts football penalties into the back of the net (for everyone except England that is) and it breaks 10 seconds for the 100 metres sprint. It is a key technique for reducing stress and anxiety so that the individual can perform to their maximum potential. The process sounds relatively simple: relax and visualise the win. However, for it to have a genuine effect learners will need support in developing the skill to shut out the negative thoughts that will prevent successful visualisations. Encourage your learner to talk through what their success will look like; this might feel a bit odd to start off with, but it is a worthwhile process as it focuses the mind on the goal very effectively.

Visualisation

Encourage your learner to visualise their success, describing and defining exactly what the success will look like and feel like. This will help focus the mind and reduce anxiety.

Self-Belief, Emotional Arousal (EA) 4: MC19

HABIT LOOPS

Habit loops are not technically part of the world of mentoring and coaching, I have actually pinched it from neuroscientific research. It has seen application to the marketing world[23] and there is some advice on using habit loops in coaching. However, it has had minimal formal impact on the coaching world, but I place it in this chapter because it has a useful application in learning conversations. When a learner needs to 'undo' bad habits in order to progress towards a specific objective, insight into their own habit loops will be invaluable. Alternatively, they may have bad learning habits that must be broken and reformed so they can develop learning skills for effective post-study learning.

Graybiel[24] has uncovered the mechanism through which the brain (the basal ganglia to be specific) utilises habitual behaviour to minimise energy expenditure in routine behaviours. Essentially the neurones in the basal ganglia have a strong positive feedback mechanism. So once a routine is embedded the relevant neurones involved will strongly attract neurotransmitters towards them as soon as the specific behaviour is initiated. This mechanism was uncovered through use of mice, mazes and a number of strategically placed electrodes. The relationship between learners and the mouse that took the right turn instead of the left is learning habits. This could be their approach to new experiences, the timings of their reflections, their preferences when looking for alternative solutions or any other part of their learning cycle that could have become unwittingly habitual. The practical applications of this are a tool to help us break unhelpful learning habits and form useful learning habits.

The research carried out by Graybiel[24] found that when a behaviour was first carried out neurones fired constantly. However, after repetition the neurones would fire at the beginning of the behaviour as the brain recognises and sources the correct habit. Then they settled down until the end of the habitual behaviour when there is a second spike in activity that provides the brain with the positive reinforcement to continue to remember this particular habit. This is the background for a habit loop: cue → habitual behaviour → reward. It gives us two points of investigation of our habits: what is the cue? And what is the reward?

If we are looking to break a bad habit we should investigate the cue for the habit and see if we can influence this is in some way. Alternatively we can look at the reward and see if there is something that we can do to remove or alter the reward so that the behaviour is not reinforced. For example, when I make my daughter a chocolate spread sandwich I have a terrible habit of helping myself to a dollop of it (I know I'm not the only one!). So what were the cues? Time of day? (Always lunchtime but not every lunchtime.) Hunger? (Not really.) My daughter's choice of sandwich filling? (Yes, but not something I can control.) Actually I realised that it was because I felt like I was running low on energy, and the reward of the psychological boost of sugar set me up for the afternoon. So now instead of eating my way through my daughter's chocolate spread I have a few grapes, which are sweet enough to trick my brain into a psychological sugar rush.

There are also situations where we need to create new learning habits. It is difficult to create a new habit from scratch because the level of repetition required to embed the new habit is high and this is likely to be time consuming and probably tedious for the learner. The good news is that it is possible to latch onto current habits and adapt or extend them to build in new behaviours. For example, one of the key challenges for many medical educators and learners is the development of reflective behaviours. Particularly since many modern training programmes require some form of reflective log. Most of us, even the worst reflectors among us, will usually find there are certain points in the week when they have a little think about events past. Rather than trying to get learners to sit down and reflect at a predetermined time each day, find out their current reflective habits and utilise the cues and rewards. For example, if they reflect while walking the dog perhaps the cue is the dog walking, so our dog-walking learner could take the dog out in the evenings after work to provoke reflective thought. Alternatively the cue could be the time of day and instead of walking the dog on a Sunday morning they should spend time completing their reflective logs. It is also worth investigating the reward for the behaviour – maybe our dog-walking learner spends Sunday afternoon with his parents-in-law and uses the time to reflect so that he has interesting topics of conversation for the afternoon.

Although we can use these ideas to guide our discussions with learners, the key is to give the learner insight into the process themselves. Without insight the learner cannot go on to use the same approach in a self-directed manner after their studies.

Habit loops

Develop an understanding of your learner's habit loops and use these to build good learning habits. Help the learner develop an understanding of their own habit loops, the cues and rewards, in order to gain insight into their learning process. They can use their deeper understanding of thought processes to improve their learning as they move forwards.

Skills, Active Experimentation (AE) 5: MC20

SUMMARY

This brings us to the end of our tour through mentoring and coaching research. We have looked at the roles of the mentor and coach, the skills needed for both and some more specific ideas from the literature that we can use to develop self-directedness. This search has uncovered 20 new bricks that could be used to build our three pillars to support self-directedness. These bricks all relate specifically to the relationship between educator and learner and trying too many at once would at the very least put a strain on the relationship. So use the overall model to identify the areas you want to work on then come back to this chapter to find the detail about those bricks that best fit your needs.

In the next chapter we will be taking a trip through research into reflective practice and action research. As was mentioned in Chapter 1, one of the criticisms of Kolb's Experiential Learning Cycle is that reflection is a single stage in the process. In Chapter 5 we will be looking in more detail at this section in particular, but we will also find lots to build our other pillars as well.

CHAPTER 5

Reflective practice and action research

'To fill our heads, like a scrapbook, with this and that item as a finished and done-for thing, is not to think. It is to turn ourselves into a piece of registering equipment.'[1] (p. 81)

INTRODUCTION

Reflection is not a new concept by any means but has risen to prominence in recent times and is now one of the cornerstones of effective learning. The modern intensification of interest is often seen as a result of Schön's key text, *Educating the Reflective Practitioner*.[2] The increased scrutiny of the reflective process has generated an increasingly complex picture of a metacognitive, self-regulatory process.[3, 4] Much of this research is highly abstract in nature and we will avoid getting caught up in the semantics in the academic world and instead we will focus on the application of these principles.

It will become clear throughout this chapter why reflective practice and action research have been placed together in a chapter (it was not just to keep the nice two topic titles for the chapters, I promise).

> Action research is one model of reflection on practice. The model is a very powerful way of orientating yourself, systematically, to the challenge of professional practice where situations are either problematic or where you feel they could be improved.[5] (p. 185)

Reflective practice manifests in different ways in medical education. For some it is an annual report by an Educational Supervisor that combines reflection with a target-setting process. For others it means completing regular reflective logs and in some cases the ability to reflect must be demonstrated through exam procedures. Unfortunately, defining it as a concept is a little tricky; it's all a bit woolly, fluffy round the edges and a little like trying to catch soap in the bath. How is reflection any different to 'just' thinking?

If we were to play a word association game and I said 'reflection', you would quite possibly reply 'mirror' (or perhaps 'pond', but that wouldn't work for this analogy). So rather than starting with a trawl through the many definitions in research let's begin with that idea. Reflection is taking a long look at yourself: your abilities, your thoughts, your values and your behaviours. It is more than just this, though, for effective reflection we need to imagine one of those unforgiving, magnifying bathroom mirrors that show up all the blemishes. However, there are limits to this analogy because it implies isolation from others, especially since I seem to have ended up in the bathroom where you tend to find me on my own. True reflective thought should include careful consideration of different perspectives as well as an honest examination of our own beliefs and actions.

There may not be a single widely accepted definition, but there are some researchers, such as Boud *et al.*[6] and Shulman,[7] who are more widely quoted than others.

> Reflection in the context of learning is a generic term for those intellectual and affective activities in which individuals engage to explore their experiences in order to lead to new understandings and appreciations. It may take place in isolation or in association with others.[6 (p. 19)]
>
> Reflection: Reviewing, reconstructing, re-enacting and critically analysing one's own … performance, and grounding explanations in evidence.[7 (p. 15)]

Part of the issue with defining reflection is the flexibility of terminology in use: is someone who is carrying out a reflective process a reflective practitioner? Does an episode of reflection, a reflective practitioner make? Is there a difference (or one that matters for us) between reflection, reflective practice, reflexive practice, critically reflecting, making reflective judgements, deliberative rationalising? This is further complicated by temporal considerations: is reflection backward looking? Forward looking? Both? Or perhaps reflection is entirely in the moment? And even worse there are individualistic considerations: do men and women think the same way? (Insert your own comment regarding multi-tasking or parking here). And what about the ever-present cultural concerns?

Among all the various muddles, perhaps the most useful thing we can do as educators is recognise the importance of reflection. To do this we need to understand the nature of reflection and develop a tacit knowledge of the reflective process. This can then be applied to our individual context and our specific learner to help them develop the reflective skills necessary for effective reflective observations of their experiences.

WHY REFLECT?

There are cries from learners everywhere of 'We don't have the time', 'It's pointless', 'It doesn't relate to the real life' and many other things that (to be frank) my editor would never allow me to put into print. So it becomes the job of the educator to sell reflection to the learner. It is very tempting to join in with them; to agree that it is a frustrating system but there are hoops we have to jump through. The problem with this is you are unlikely to get 'buy in' from the learner, which will probably mean one or both of two things. First, the learner may not complete the necessary reflections because they do not see anyone visibly and believably enforcing the requirement. Second, they may not actually improve their reflective skills as any reflection carried out is too shallow to be effective. So let us first look at three key reasons to get on board with reflection.

Probably Schön's biggest, or certainly most well-known, contribution to reflective practice literature was his concept of reflection-in-action and reflection-on-action.[2] There is not actually a significant amount of evidence to support this division of reflection into 'in action' and 'on action'.[8] However, the breadth of the acceptance by educationalists and the ease with which people integrate the idea into their practice indicates that it clearly strikes a chord for those on the educational front line. Reflection-in-action is those tiny adjustments that we make: when we drive a car we constantly adjust the direction and speed of the car to compensate for wind, hills, the car in front and such like. This ongoing process of reflection can be difficult to dissect because much of it would fall into the 'unknown known' so it can be difficult to demonstrate it to learners.

> While a professional is consciously aware of the knowledge used while reflecting-on-action, this may not be so for reflection-in-action, and therefore it may be difficult for practitioners to articulate the knowledge they are using in action.[9 (p. 1188)]

Instead, we can use the reflection-on-action process that happens after the event as an entrance point to the learner's ability to reflect. The skills that the learner develops when reflecting-on-action will be internalised and will become part of the reflection-in-action process. In Chapter 4 we discussed the usefulness of Graybiel's[10] work on habit loops and introduced the idea that reflection can become habitual. In the context of Schön's model we are 'habitualising' reflection-on-action in order to ensure that habitual reflection-in action is effective and insightful. So the first selling point for encouraging reflection is the access it provides to the skills needed for ongoing adjustments made during practice.

Second, reflection is important as part of a continual process of challenge towards our assumptions and rationalisations. Brookfield[11] discusses the work by King and Kitchener[12] (see later for more on their work) and describes how important it is to challenge the underlying reasoning for the beliefs we hold.

> Learning how to learn involves an epistemological awareness deeper than simply knowing how one scores on a cognitive style inventory, or what is one's typical or preferred pattern of learning. Rather, it means that adults possess a self-conscious awareness of how it is they come to know what they know; an awareness of the reasoning, assumptions, evidence and justifications that underlie our beliefs that something is true.[11]

Cognitive theories hold that our beliefs form the foundation for our thoughts, which in turn construct our actions. Therefore if we wish to affect our actions we must challenge our beliefs.

Mezirow[13] discusses the categorisations that we all make, sometimes known (often with negative connotations) as stereotyping. These categorisations are initially based upon limited experiences; we make generalisations that allow us to predict and hypothesise future events (think back to Kelly's constructivism discussed in Chapter 3). This may not be a problem and may, in fact, help us to manage the daily onslaught of information. However, problems arise when we perceive only the information that supports our generalisation, when only the bits of reality that meet the expectations of the stereotype are 'seen'. The generalisation is reinforced, resulting in invalid assumptions because the perceived reality is incomplete.

Loughran[14] emphasises the importance of the difference between rationalisation, justification and reflection.

> One might justify practice in terms of a particular way of approaching a situation because of specific knowledge or thoughts about that setting; however, rationalization is the dogged adherence to an approach almost despite the nature of the practice setting because alternative ways of seeing are not (cannot) be apprehended.[14 (p. 35)]

Justification is to some extent a defence mechanism. In the real world it is not always possible for all actions to be congruent with values. Therefore, we make justifications that there is a particular reason for this mismatch that is out of our control: 'It's in the guidelines', 'It is how the senior nurse likes it done', 'It is the only way I can actually find time to treat all my patients.' These justifications are important for us to continue in the face of a reality that does not allow us to always meet our own expectations. However, if these become too engrained they become rationalisations that are resistant to change. This can be especially tricky if a negative experience triggered the reflection.

> Negative feelings disturb us and are played out as anxiety. People are strongly moti-
> vated to resolve anxiety through the use of defence mechanisms. As such, people
> may naturally reflect to defend against anxiety rather than to learn through it. I
> use the word reflect loosely because in this sense it does not lead to insight. It is
> an effort to deal with the consequence of a situation rather than its causes.[15] (p. 43)

So the second reason to explicitly work to improve reflective skills is to ensure beliefs, assumptions and generalisations are challenged. Genuine reflection prevents justifications becoming rationalisations and does not allow us to make excuses to ourselves when we have had a negative experience.

Finally, healthcare is an emotional arena to work in. In some cases this emotion has to be contained: a surgeon needs a certain amount of detachment if they are to take a knife to their patient. At the other extreme are those who use their emotions as a tool to help them empathise with the patient to deal with them in a holistic manner. In either case, it is very important that the learner puts aside some time to reflect upon these emotions.[8] Learners should attempt to understand them from a cognitive perspective – to work through exactly why they are experiencing these emotions, what it is about their situation and past experiences that affect their perceptions and responses to the events. A deeper understanding of their emotions will help learners develop emotional coping strategies. Learners need the ability to manage their emotions on a day to day basis because it will be difficult for a learner to move forward when they are feeling dragged down by an emotive work situation. The stress and anxiety induced will lower their belief that they would be capable of achieving a task.

Emotional reflection

Make sure learners understand the importance of reflecting on their emotions and analysing the root causes of their feelings towards their experiences. A better understanding of previous negative emotional responses will help the learner feel more able to make repeat attempts.

Self-belief, Emotional Arousal (EA) 5: RA1

There is a tendency for reflection to be prompted by negative emotions; however, it is sometimes useful to reflect on positive feelings. This is especially relevant in the context of self-directedness: by reflecting on positive experiences learners will be emphasising their successes.

> Reflection is often triggered by negative or uncomfortable feelings. As such, models of reflection draw the user's attention to feelings. It seems natural to focus on negative experiences because it is these situations that present themselves to consciousness. Much of experience is not reflected on simply because it is unproblematic. In other words, much of experience is taken for granted.[15 (p. 43)]

Positive reflection

Encourage your learner to reflect on positive experiences as well as negative. There is much to be learned from analysing how and why something went well and learners will be buoyed by their achievements.

Self-belief, Performance Accomplishments, (PA) 5: RA2

LEVELS OF REFLECTION

There are several scales that describe in varying detail the different levels of reflection. Some are simple scales that are related directly to learning to like surface processing and deep processing (such as Dinsmore and Alexander[16]) or single loop and double loop learning (Argyris and Schön[17]). These models describe the learning that happens as a result of a deep understanding of the problem and the context. Many of the more complex models are rooted in the developmental ideas proposed by Piaget,[18] so the levels are seen as consecutive and a learner progresses through them as they age and mature. However, the higher levels of reflectivity described are unlikely to be achieved by most without some form of support and guidance. We will take a look at two of these age-related approaches: Mezirow[13] and King and Kitchener.[12]

Mezirow

Mezirow[13] based his studies of reflectivity within the context of the three cognitive interests proposed by Habermas:[19] technical, practical and emancipatory. These are linked to three areas of social interest: work, interaction and power respectively. Mezirow's work is focused on the third of these areas: emancipatory.

> This involves an interest in self-knowledge, that is, the knowledge of self-reflection, including interest in the way one's history and biography has expressed itself in the way one sees oneself, one's roles and social expectations. Emancipation is from libidinal, institutional or environmental forces which limit our options and rational control over our lives but have been taken for granted as beyond human control. Insights gained through critical self-awareness are emancipatory in the sense that at least one can recognise the correct reasons for his or her problems.[13 (p. 5)]

Emancipation is a fundamental consideration in developing self-directedness. Learners who assume that surrounding forces are out of their control and have no awareness of their own part in them may feel constrained in their learning. When the learner makes choices for future learning they can easily lay blame for lack of engagement or missed opportunities with these external forces. So built in to Mezirow's model of reflectivity is the concept of perspective transformation which is inextricably linked to the adult education principle of transformational learning. It is the process of the learner becoming critically aware of how they perceive their reality, their thoughts and their actions as well as their habits that are associated with each of these. The learner develops an understanding of the cultural assumptions they are making, where cultural means both the immediate culture within which they are working and learning and the wider cultural influences that will be exerted upon them. This process of perspective transformation will be key to the development of self-directedness.

> A self-directed learner must be understood as one who **is aware of the constraints on his efforts to learn**, including the **psycho-cultural assumptions** involving reified **power relationships** embedded in **institutionalised ideologies** which influence one's habits of perception, thought and behaviour as one attempts to learn. A self-directed learner has **access to alternative perspectives** for understanding his or her situation and for giving meaning and direction to his or her life, has **acquired sensitivity and competence in social interaction** and has the skills and competences required to master the productive tasks associated with **controlling and manipulating the environment**.[13 (p. 21)]

You may want to go back and read that last quote again. It really is worth internalising.

Mezirow provides three objects for reflecting upon: the learner's perceptions, thoughts and actions (*see* Figure 5.1). Associated with each of these are the habits that the learner will have formed because they will respond habitually to environmental stimuli. Mezirow's model describes two overall modes of reflectivity: conscious and critically conscious, each of which has a number of sub-levels. In the conscious modes of reflectivity there are four sub-levels.

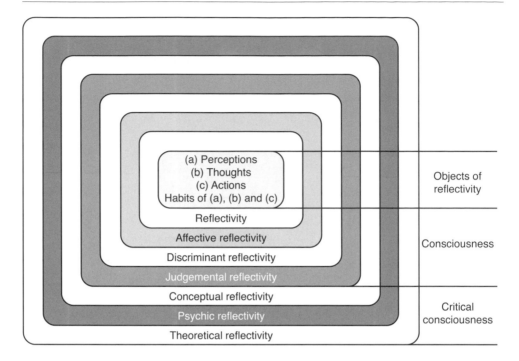

FIGURE 5.1 Mezirow's model of reflectivity

- Reflectivity: learners develop a simple awareness of a specific perception, thought, action and/or habit.
- Affective reflectivity: learners develop an awareness of the feelings associated with the perception, thought, action and/or habit.
- Discriminant reflectivity: learners begin to assess the efficacy of their perceptions, thoughts, actions and habits. They begin to understand the root causes of these and the reality of the context they operate in and the relationships that they have formed.
- Judgemental reflectivity: learners develop an awareness of value judgements (or lack thereof) about their perceptions, thoughts, actions and habits. Learners begin to judge whether or not these are positive or negative aspects of themselves.

Each level is seen as incorporating the previous levels so this is a progressive scale. The next mode of reflectivity, critical consciousness, involves meta-learning and has a further three sub-levels.

- Conceptual reflectivity: the learner begins to question whether their concepts of, for example, 'good' and 'bad' are adequate for making judgements. They begin to reflect on how their own judgements are formed and challenge whether they are appropriate, fair or stringent enough to judge others and their actions as well as their own.

- Psychic reflectivity: the learner identifies their own tendencies to form snap judgements about people (and ideas) on the basis of little or biased information.
- Theoretical reflectivity: the learner recognises that the reason they make snap judgements is because they have not got a deep enough awareness of the cultural influences exerted upon them. They understand that they have a single perspective that is not necessarily the best for viewing a situation. Their deeply engrained psychological assumptions based upon personal experiences are recognised and the learner realises that they do not necessarily hold the whole picture.

Theoretical reflectivity is the level of reflectivity that forms the central process for perspective transformation. While there is not a direct link between the development of these levels and age or maturity Mezirow sees critical reflectivity, and especially theoretical reflectivity, as an adult skill that is a fundamental part of adult learning.

Mezirow moves on to discuss the difficulties of 'teaching' reflectivity. The first of Habermas' learning domains (technical) is relatively easily dealt with through learning objectives and needs analysis. However, the second (practical – social interactions) and the third (emancipation) are not so easily achieved. He suggests that learners need to be led to a position from which they can critically reflect upon their own judgement processes, the cultural influences, and assumptions and generalisations that they carry with them.

> [Learners] 'must be led to an understanding of the reasons imbedded in these internalised cultural myths and concomitant feelings which account for their felt needs and wants as well as the way they see themselves and their relations. Having gained this understanding, learners must be given access to alternative meaning perspectives for interpreting this reality so that critique of these psycho-cultural assumptions is possible.[13 (p. 18)]

Mezirow describes four mechanisms that educators can use to help them develop a perspective transformation approach.
- Work outwards from the learner perspective and develop pictures and stories that demonstrate the alternative perspectives. Pose hypothetical situations which challenge the learners to reconsider their own assumptions and reflect on the basis for their perceptions, thoughts and actions. Challenge any aspect of the context of the reflection that you feel the learner is taking for granted. Focus on the 'meta-learning' not the immediate context wherever possible. Initially learners are usually unaccustomed to being challenged at this level; they expect to be asked about the differential diagnosis. However, given time they will begin to develop the higher level reflectivity skills described by Mezirow.

- Use small groups to challenge the basis for learners' reflections perhaps through problem-based learning style scenarios. Learners will be able to draw on the experiences and perspectives of their peers as a direct challenge to their own experiences and perspectives.
- Personalise the learning: 'critical reflectivity is fostered with a premium placed on personalising what is learned by applying insights to one's own life and works as opposed to mere intellectualisation'.[13 (p. 19)]
- A process known as 'breaching' in which the educator steps back from the traditional information-giver/activity organiser role. In this case the learners are left to their own devices (within reason of course) and the educator becomes a resource for them to draw on as required. Again, this may initially be an uncomfortable situation for learners who are used to structure, but with guidance they can reflect on the reasons they feel unsettled and learn more about themselves.
- Finally, the educator can use T groups as a mechanism for developing perspective transformations. These are unstructured but facilitated meetings in which participants share emotions in an open and non-judgemental forum.

Critical reflection

Learners' critical reflective skills will likely begin as simple, surface processes where they acknowledge the issues and are aware of their feelings but spend little time challenging or analysing their thought processes. Support them to develop these skills through perspective transformation, encourage learners to see their own thoughts as a result of the wider environment and temporal contexts. A genuine understanding of the bigger picture is a very motivating experience in its own right.

Motivation, Self-Transcendence (ST) 2: RA3

King and Kitchener

King and Kitchener[12] examined hundreds of reflective conversations with individuals from adolescence to adulthood and identified seven progressive stages. They laid out descriptors for each of the seven stages and called it the Reflective Judgement Model. Their background is critical thinking and as such these stages are tied to wider critical thinking processes as well as reflective thinking.

- **Stage 1:** Knowing is limited to single concrete observations: what a person observes is true.
- **Stage 2:** Two categories for knowing: right and wrong answers. Good authorities have knowledge; bad authorities lack knowledge.

- **Stage 3:** In some areas, knowledge is certain and authorities have that knowledge. In other areas, knowledge is temporarily uncertain. Only personal beliefs can be known.
- **Stage 4:** The concept that knowledge is unknown in several specific cases leads to the abstract generalisation that knowledge is uncertain.
- **Stage 5:** Knowledge is uncertain and must be understood within a context; thus justification is context specific.
- **Stage 6:** Knowledge is uncertain but constructed by comparing evidence and opinion on different sides of an issue or across contexts.
- **Stage 7:** Knowledge is the outcome of a process of reasonable inquiry. This view is equivalent to a general principle that is consistent across domains.[12] (p. 31)

Deep reflective processes

Help your learner understand how to deepen their reflective processes through an understanding of the levels of reflection and through questioning in reflective discussions. This is a key skill for healthcare workers who must continue to learn throughout their career, often from real experiences and informal learning situations.

Skills, Reflective Observation (RO) 5: RA4

THE REFLECTIVE PROCESS

Before we embark upon this brief review of approaches to the reflective process, I am going to add a health warning:

> I must emphasise that all models of reflection are merely devices to help the practitioner to access reflection; they are not a prescription of what reflection is. Put another way, models are heuristic – a means towards an end, not an end in itself.[15] (p. 36)

Or alternatively:

> The model is not the reality; it aims to represent the reality.[20] (p. 27)

Reflection is a personal process and for many it will not follow any of the logical staged approaches laid out below. These are a starting point, somewhere to begin the process and a way to remember the different aspects to reflection. Different individuals will identify with different approaches and, as an educator, you will need a variety of reflective tools to help different learners and you will need to be prepared to flex with different learners and different situations. It is more important to achieve depth of reflection than to have a nice orderly conversation. Although it may be useful towards the end of any reflective conversation to utilise something like the processes described below to summarise and gain coherence to a learner's thoughts, don't let these models constrain an otherwise productive conversation.

Reflection as a cycle

There are many cycles that describe the reflective process, and interestingly most are not 'just' the reflective stage but also include more forward-thinking stages of action plans and changes to future practice. This is perhaps representative of the issues of reflection as a standalone tool. There is a risk that reflection without application to the future would result in a backward-looking learner. To avoid this many models of the reflective process are practically orientated and embedded in actual experience; they take the new knowledge from reflective thoughts and move forwards from there.

Gibbs[21] has produced one of the most well-known reflective cycles. It is firmly grounded in experiential learning, which squares nicely with our first pillar of self-directedness. Gibbs describes how his cycle fits into the Experiential Learning Cycle as reflections must be based upon meaningful experiences for the learner.

> Openness to experience is necessary for learners to have the evidence upon which to reflect. It is therefore crucial to establish an appropriate emotional tone for learners: one which is safe and supportive, and which encourages learners to value their own experience and to trust themselves to draw conclusions from it. This openness may not exist at the outset but may be fostered through successive experiences of the experiential learning cycle.[21 (p. 15)]

The 'reality' of the experience provided can be placed along a spectrum of different types of experience that a learner may encounter in their training (*see* Figure 5.2).

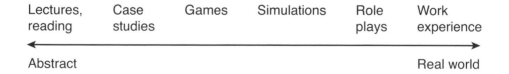

FIGURE 5.2 Types of experience

> ## Reality of experience
>
> Reflection can result from a variety of different experiences that range from real experience, through role plays, simulations, games and case studies to lectures and reading. As the learning experience becomes more realistic, the potential quality of reflection also increases. Providing these real world experiences will give our learners better opportunities to learn and to practise their learning skills.
>
> *Skills, Concrete Experience (CE) 6: RA5*

Gibbs developed a reflective cycle (*see* Figure 5.3) as a tool for educators to use to guide learners through debriefing sessions. The sequence of steps suggests a series of thought exercises before embarking upon the action planning stage of the cycle.

1. Description: What happened? Don't make judgements at this stage or try to draw conclusions; simply describe.
2. Feelings: What were your reactions and feelings? Again don't move on to analysing these yet.
3. Evaluation: What was good or bad about the experience? Make value judgements.
4. Analysis: What sense can you make of the situation? Bring in ideas from outside the experience to help you. What was really going on? Were different people's experiences similar or different in important ways?
5. Conclusions (general): What can be concluded, in a general sense, from these experiences and analyses you have undertaken?
6. Conclusions (specific): What can be concluded about your own specific, unique, personal situation or way of working?
7. Personal action plans: What are you going to do different (if anything) in this type of situation next time? What steps are you going to take on the basis of what you have learnt?[21] (pp. 32–3)

This cycle divides facts from feelings and it separates the analytical, judgemental thoughts that often come naturally to us. It is common for the judging process to begin before the learner has undertaken genuine fact finding and identified their associated feelings. By holding these judgemental thoughts back the learner can form judgements based on better information.

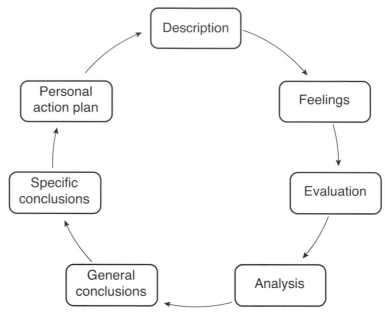

FIGURE 5.3 Gibbs' reflective cycle

Reflection as a series of questions

Borton[22] put forward the well-known 'What? So what? Now what?' structure for reflective discussions, and the simplicity of this approach is perhaps at the root of its popularity. Further detail was added by Driscoll[23] that provides more depth to the three stages:

1. A description of the event: What? trigger question.
   What is the purpose of returning to this situation?
   What happened?
   What did I see/do?
   What was my reaction to it?
   What did other people who were involved do?
2. An analysis of the event: So What? trigger questions.
   How did I feel at the time of the event?
   Were those feelings I had any different from those of other people who were also involved at the time?
   Are my feelings now, after the event, any different from what I experienced at the time?
   Do I still feel troubled, if so, in what way?
   What were the effects of what I did (or did not do)?
   What positive aspects now emerge for me from the event that happened in practice?

What have I noticed about my behaviour in practice by taking a more measured look at it?

What observations does any person helping me to reflect on my practice make of the way I acted at the time?

3. Proposed actions following the event: Now What? trigger questions.

What are the implications for me, and others in clinical practice, based on what I have described and analysed?

What difference does it make if I choose to do nothing?

Where can I get more information to face a similar situation again?

How could I modify my practice if a similar situation was to happen again?

What support do I need to help me 'action' the results of my reflections?

Which aspect should be tackled first?

How will I notice that I am any different in clinical practice?

What is the main learning that I take from reflecting on my practice in this way?[23] (p. 45)

The length of this list means that (unless they have a very good memory) the educator would need to keep a crib sheet nearby. Sitting with a list of questions on your lap is unlikely to bring about an atmosphere conducive to reflection; after all we don't want our learners to feel like they are being interviewed. However, we can still use them as prompts to help flesh out the simple three step process described by Borton.

The reflective conversation

Have a number of strategies in your toolkit to help guide reflective conversations and share these with the learner. This will improve the structure of reflective discussions and help learners to develop the skills to reflect in a manner that provides relevant targets and action plans.

Skills, Reflective Observation (RO) 6: RA6

ENCOURAGING REFLECTION

Some learners will be naturally reflective in their approach while others will find this aspect of learning very difficult. Honey and Mumford[24] identified four learning preferences: activist, theorist, pragmatist and reflector. Educators working with those learners who have a low natural preference for reflection will need a toolkit of useful techniques to help learners develop their reflective skills. What follows is a brief selection of these tools (taken from Thompson and Thompson[25]) that could prove useful in developing the reflective skills needed for our self-directed learners to learn through experience.

- Three Hs: Head, Heart and Habit

  These three 'H' words provide a prompt that encourages the reflector to consider the source of their thoughts. Are their instinctive reactions the result of their head, their heart or their habits? It is important that these three H's are aligned in any action plan, as this is the best way to ensure that the planned approach will proceed effectively and lead to success.

The 3 H's

When reflecting on situations and setting targets with a learner, consider where the origin of their thoughts lie: in their head, their heart or as a result of habitual thoughts and actions. This analysis will help learners ensure their head, heart and habits are congruent with one another as they plan the way forward increasing the chances of success.

Self-belief, Performance Accomplishments (PA) 6: RA7

- The CIA framework

  The CIA framework: Control, Influence, Acceptance, is useful for reflection on stressful events or problems that are causing significant concern to the learner. In all circumstances there are always some factors we can control, some that we can influence and some that we can neither control nor influence that we must simply accept.

The CIA framework

Learners will often find it hard to deal with the emotions involved in a job in health-care and sometimes it falls to the educator to help them move past this. Analysing their situation by considering which factors they can control, which they can influence and which they must accept will help bring the matter into clarity. If the learner can truly accept that there are aspects out of their control they will be able to relax more, so putting them in a better position to take risks with their learning.

Self-belief, Emotional Arousal (EA) 6: RA8

- The objectives tree (*see* Figure 5.4)

  This approach does not initially appear particularly reflective; however, it is useful to help develop a reflective approach to the planning process. It encourages clear thinking related to the factors needed for success and how these can be achieved in a very stepwise and visual manner. There are three questions which form three layers to the tree: What are you trying to achieve? What factors will contribute to the success of this? What actions are needed to make sure these factors contribute to a successful outcome? These three questions are laid out in a tree configuration.

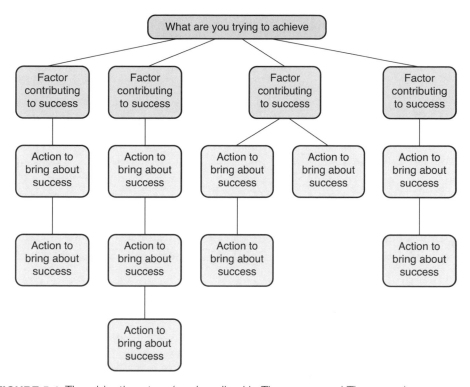

FIGURE 5.4 The objectives tree (as described in Thompson and Thompson)

The objectives tree

Taking a structured reflective approach to planning that considers the many facets that could lead to success and the specific actions required to make these come about will increase the chances of success. The learner that feels they have successfully planned and achieved is going to feel an increased level of self-efficacy, improving the likelihood they will embark upon future opportunities with confidence.

Self-belief, Performance Accomplishments (PA) 7: RA9

REFLECTING ON YOURSELF AS AN EDUCATOR

It would be inappropriate to move on without considering the reflectivity of the educator themselves. As will be discussed in Chapter 6, modelling forms a substantial part of encouraging best practice and therefore educators should be demonstrating their own reflections in the educational context and, where appropriate, in the workplace context.

> An effective way to improve the quality of reflective discussion is to provide a direct experience of what such a discussion can be like by 'modelling'. Modelling is simply providing a clear model or example, and shaping learners' behaviour towards this model.[21] (p. 35)

Van Manen[26] developed three levels of reflectivity or 'deliberative rationality', specifically for educators to reflect upon the learning environment.

1. Educators operating at the first level tend to reflect on how the teaching went rather than on whether any learning actually took place. They may reflect upon the use of some basic educational principles, but only with reference to how these were applied, not whether they were effective in improving learning. The choice of which educational principles to use is based upon a pragmatic approach where the most efficient option is selected. Once the educator realises they are operating within these constraints it opens the door for them to access a higher level of reflectivity.

2. At level two, educational choices are assumed to be based upon a predetermined set of educational values belonging to whoever designed the course or curriculum. Reflective processes accept these as a given and apply it to practical experience. Educators reflecting at this level will recognise the learning and the learner as a key part of the educational process in which educators and learners find themselves in a partnership. If, however, educators begin to challenge the prevailing values of the curriculum or course and embed their reflections into the learner's perspective, they will begin to reflect at Van Manen's highest level of reflectivity.

3. At level three the reflecting educator is constantly challenging the reasoning behind the choice of learning objectives and the methodology used to achieve it. Knowledge is placed within social contexts in order to ensure their relevance for learners and reflection focuses on how effectively this was achieved. The usefulness of the knowledge being delivered is consistently reviewed by the educator as they remain open minded to the worth (or not) of the content of the learning and the teaching strategies employed. Educators recognise the importance of the relationship with the learner and much of their reflection will be upon where the balance of the relationship lies.

Shulman[7] studied the reflective processes of teachers. He identified four knowledge bases for teachers.

1. Knowledge of the course content and of different ways of knowing this information. Teachers should also be aware of critical literature associated with this knowledge.
2. Knowledge of the curriculum, assessments and other educational materials and structures.
3. Knowledge of the processes of teaching and of learning.
4. Knowledge of the ongoing process of teaching; the educator learns through experiences and is able to fluidly adjust to different contexts. This is called the wisdom of practice.

These sources of knowledge form the possible areas for educators to acquire new comprehensions. Shulman suggests that the new constructs formed from these four sources of knowledge can form the basis for a reflective process.

Modelling reflective practice

Educators should model effective reflective practice and openly demonstrate the reflective process. Dissect your own reflection-in-action and reflection-on-action and recognise your own strengths and weaknesses in the skill of reflection. This allows learners to see that the process is both achievable but also an ongoing process of improvement. The impact will be even better if this can be achieved through group work with their peers.

Self-belief, Vicarious Experiences (VE) 3: RA10

ACTION RESEARCH

In the varied topography of professional practice, there is a high, hard ground overlooking a swamp. On the high ground, manageable problems lend themselves to solution through the application of research-based theory and technique. In the swampy lowland, messy, confusing problems defy technical solutions. The irony of this situation is that the problems of the high ground tend to be relatively unimportant to individuals or society at large, however great their technical interest may be, while in the swamp lie the problems of greatest human concern. The practitioner must choose. Shall he remain on the high ground where he can problem solve relatively unimportant problems according to prevailing standards of rigor, or shall he descend to the swamp of important problems and non-rigorous enquiry?[2] (p. 3)

This quote from Schön[2] poses a question: is it really a choice between the highlands and the lowlands? I do not think so. In modern day education that threshold between theory and practice has blurred and a lot of research is now positioned to provide directly applicable, practical information. There is much to be gained for an individual to repeatedly cross the border between the highlands and the swamp. Get a taste of theory from the highlands then enter the lowlands, try it out, adapt it but keep it fundamentally grounded in what is currently evidenced as best practice. After a while hike back up from the swamp to the highlands and dip into a little more theory, find out new information and keep up to date with evidence-based education. It does not have to be a choice. While 'the problems of real-world practice do not present themselves to practitioners as well-formed problems',[2 (p. 4)] this is not a reason to completely abandon the highlands.

Interestingly, Schön identified a need for research to get a bit messier and this indeed happened very soon after he published the above quote. This 'messy' form of research (enthusiasts will not appreciate me calling it messy but please hang on in there) was called action research. There is some controversy over where the action research movement began – in the highlands or the lowlands – but either way the process provides a personalised bridge between generalised theory and the individual's practice.

Around the 1940s the educational research world began to undergo a paradigm shift. There was a gradual acceptance of qualitative research accompanied by a realisation that there is not a single truth to be sought but multiple truths for multiple contexts. Action research has arisen as part of this 'new' research.

> [Action research emphasises] the idea of knowledge generation as creative practice that evolves through dialogue. It recognises knowledge not only as an outcome of cognitive activity, but also as embodied; that is, mind and body are not perceived as separate entities but as integrated. Knowledge is arrived at, and exists in, feeling and multiple sensory modes. Consequently knowledge exists as much 'in here' as 'out there'.[20 (p. 117)]

Now I know that the scientist in us may be jumping about shouting 'wishy-washy stuff, the hypothesis is objective, the researcher is a neutral observer', but read on just a bit more. Action research is not about finding the one answer, just as cancer research is not about the cure for cancer. It recognises that just as we cannot group together all cancers for one cure, we cannot group all educators, learners, contexts and find a single educational 'cure'. If we accept this as the case, and I think we must, it becomes difficult to imagine that educational research should not be heavily context driven including both internal, personal contexts and wider, external contexts. It is the same premise that forms the basis for the third layer of our model of self-directedness; there is not a 'magic bullet', instead there are a number of evidence-based bricks that can be put together to make up our three pillars in whichever way best suits your context. Hart and Bond[27] identify seven criteria of action research which quite clearly describe the nature of action research. It:

1. is educative
2. deals with individuals as members of social groups
3. is problem-focused, context specific and future-orientated;
4. involves a change intervention;
5. aims at improvement and involvement;
6. involves a cyclic process in which research, action and evaluation are interlinked;
7. is founded on a research relationship in which those involved are participants in the change process.[27 (pp. 37–8)]

Asking the right questions for action research

The question the researcher poses for action research is one of the fundamental differences between action research and other more traditional forms of research. The question is about 'me', 'my context', 'my improvement'. That is not to say action research is a selfish act, far from it; it is a constantly reviewed process of self-improvement for the benefit of others as much as for oneself.

Since the question for action research stems from the individual it has to be related to that individual; it is not a hunt for a hypothesis that can tested to determine whether it is true or false. The stimulus for the question may stem from an unsatisfactory tutorial or negative relationship with a learner that provides an obvious avenue for exploration through action research. Alternatively, we may use internal reflections to direct our wish to improve. Whitehall[28] suggests we are looking for something in our practice that makes us feel uncomfortable.

> … the incentive for beginning a personal study to come from experiencing oneself as a 'living contradiction'; that is, feeling dissonance when we are not acting in accordance with our values and beliefs.[20 (p. 59)]

Action research questions may begin 'How do I …?', 'How can I …?', 'What would happen if I …?'. In each case, the question relates to the individual researcher. The action research question associated with this book would be 'How do I encourage my learner to be self-directed?' And here is the bit that will really upset those whose concept of research is fully embedded in the traditional, scientific approach: the question is not carved in stone. It is perfectly acceptable to come back to the question part way through the research and change it. Again and again. There is little point continuing to research a particular question relevant to the individual if the data collection exposes a variant that is more relevant.

THE ACTION RESEARCH PROCESS

With the question decided, the research process can begin. We have already identified the question as one of the key differences between action research and traditional research but what is the difference between action research and 'self-improvement'? The answer lies in the collection of evidence. It is probably relatively common for us to find an area for improvement then, with a bit of reflection and maybe asking some advice, we get on and make a change. But the challenge is what this change is based on. Did we make sure we fully understood the initial context? Our own values? The people and environmental factors involved? Did we consider our problem in the context of evidence from research? If not we are probably proceeding with little more than a hunch, hoping that we have the right instincts and that the change will actually work. You never know, maybe it will, but even if it does

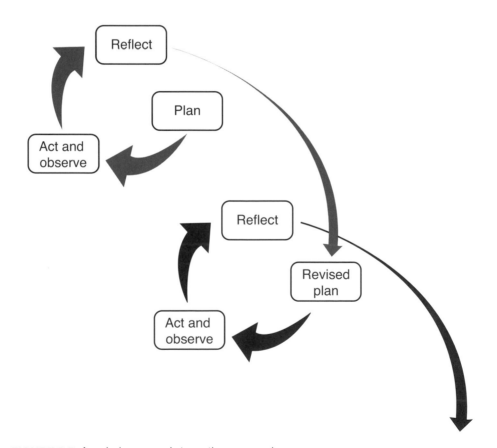

FIGURE 5.5 A spiral approach to action research

we may never fully understand why it worked or be able to replicate it in the future. Action research is more rigorous than this: it involves collecting and triangulating data through authentic descriptive accounts, qualitative counts, videos and observations. This initial process may seem to frustratingly delay a change to our practice, but it is what sets action research apart from 'wishy-washy'. Kemmis and McTaggart[29] describe a spiral process of planning (data collection, question finding), acting and observing (continuous monitoring) and reflecting (evaluating) (*see* Figure 5.5). This feeds into a revised plan which is actioned, observed and reflected upon and so on.

The problem is that in the 'messy' educational context, each stage of the process may uncover other elements of practice for consideration. The trick to successful action research is to identify those factors that need to be considered in the current cycle and those that are simply drawing you away from the actual target for improvement.

Many approaches to action research, like that described above, depersonalise the process, which is slightly counterintuitive because it is an inherently personal process. Whitehead[28] suggests five questions which view the process from the researcher's perspective. He identified a five-step method that emphasises the individual and potentially personal nature of this type of research. The questions describe how the process feels to the individual:

1. I experience a problem when some of my educational values are negated in my practice
2. I imagine a solution to my problem
3. I act in the direction of the solution
4. I evaluate the outcomes of my actions
5. I modify my problems, ideas and actions in the light of my evaluations.

I think that there is an additional and important stage to be added between steps one and two: 'I research other people's solutions to similar problems'. In my experience we are often guilty of reinventing the wheel and even though the context is king in action research it is still sensible to look at the solutions that others have tried. We all put lots of effort into finding solutions to problems that are faced by educators up and down the country and in doing so we may be wasting time and energy and risk missing out on the best solution. There also needs to be a little caution with the wording 'imagine a solution' because Whitehead is not intending the solution to appear out of thin air. Instead the solution is created after a great deal of data collection.

The action research process is closely linked with Kolb's Experiential Learning Cycle,[30] which is hardly surprising as the roots for both concepts can be found in the work of Kurt Lewin. Many of the skills practised in carrying out action research will help our learners to develop an approach of continuous improvement.

The educator as action researcher

As an educator you have a responsibility to your learners to be open to new ideas and continually working through a process of self-improvement. Utilising an action research approach for this self-improvement will not only provide additional rigour and success to your own improvements but will also prove important in demonstrating the process to learners. When they see their educators working towards personal goals in a rigorous manner they are more likely to take on this approach in their own practice.

Self-belief, Vicarious Experience (VE) 4: RA11

The learner as action researcher

Educate your learners about the action research process and encourage them to use it throughout their training and beyond. It is essentially a rigorous methodology for self-directed learning that helps them link evidence, data and theory to their day to day practice. Incorporating an evidence and theory-based approach into their learning cycle will make it a more rigorous and valid process.

Skills, Abstract Conceptualisation (AC) 4: RA12

CRITICISMS OF ACTION RESEARCH

Although I have no wish to get bogged down in the academic debate of what constitutes 'true' action research, it would be unbalanced to not add in a note from detractors from the action research movement.

TABLE 5.1 The nature of and criticisms of action research

The nature of action research	The resultant issue
Personal and aligned with individual beliefs	The researcher has a vested interest in the outcome – significant potential for bias
Can be carried out by anyone	The researcher is often learning methodologies as they go – leading to poorly planned methods
Specific to context	Not always generalizable
Ties the educator and context together	Research often done among the hustle of everyday routine, which can lead to a lack of rigour in the execution of methodologies

Most objections stem from issues with the overall validity of the research and whether the methodology is rigorous enough for high-quality academic research. The challenge lies in making the reflection honest and open; the analysis must be thorough or the subsequent changes and evaluations are invalid.

Many of the identified problems with action research are linked to its fundamental nature (*see* Table 5.1). However, this discussion regarding the academic rigour of action research does risk dragging the approach up into the highlands of academia too far from the swampy lowlands to be of use to educators. Zeichner[31] describes why, perhaps, these arguments do not really matter for those of us in the lowlands.

> When I use the term 'action research', I am using it in a very broad sense as a systematic inquiry by practitioners about their own practices. There has been a lot of debate in the literature about what is and is not real action research, about the specifics of the action research spiral, about whether action research must be collaborative or not, about whether it can or should involve outsiders as well as insiders, and so on. ... A lot of this discourse, although highly informative in an academic sense, is essentially irrelevant to many of those who actually engage in action research.[31 (p. 200)]

It is for the individual to decide how far they want to take these considerations of rigour and validity when carrying out their own action research cycles. For many educators the general process will be enough to produce significant evidence-based improvements in practice. The methodology is a means to improvement rather than a publishable endpoint, although of course the more action research that is published the greater the resource set available for other practitioners. Share the good practice rather than reinvent the wheel. Again. The sharing of good practice is fundamental to the educational world, and we can learn a lot about what works (and what doesn't) in contexts similar to our own to help us generate suitable goals and solutions. Sharing successes allows the teaching and learning process to continually evolve as patterns are identified across contexts. We can then use our own expertise to translate these generalisations into our day to day practice.

SUMMARY

This concludes our hunt through the research into reflective practice and the action research process. The development of reflective skills is so important in the healthcare environment and yet it is still one that presents one of the biggest challenges. Utilising some of the ideas presented here is a starting point to overcome this challenge, whether this is through the quick reflective tips or the broader action research approach.

In our next chapter we will study research into learning and teaching, which is an obvious area for us to find a large number of bricks to help build our pillars of self-directedness. As we begin the next chapter keep in mind that we are, as with the whole book, looking to improve the learners' insight into the process as much as we are seeking to improve our own teaching. Ultimately, improving our teaching is about improving learning and prompting transformational moments for our learners as they develop insight into their learning process.

CHAPTER 6

Learning and teaching

'Anyone who stops learning is old, whether at twenty or eighty. Anyone who keeps learning stays young.'

attributed to Henry Ford

Perhaps inevitably our search for supporting literature moves into the world of learning and teaching (after many years of the phrase being teaching and learning someone, somewhere decided that actually the learning should be first since it is the most important). Much of this research is based on education for children; however, we will not discount these ideas simply because they originated in the school classroom. Knowles[1] argued that pedagogy (educating children) and andragogy (educating adults) are separate entities because adults required a more experiential, problem-solving approach. However, Knowles was writing at a time when primary and secondary teaching was still, for the majority, didactic and passive in nature. Anyone with children in school will realise that this is no longer the case (for the majority). Therefore, the context has changed and there is a significant movement within education that believes the differences between child and adult learning are minimal. The reasoning is two-fold: first, children also benefit from active, experiential, problem-based learning and, second, andragogy assumes that all adults are the same and have reached a maturation that automatically differentiates them from children.

There is a lot of research and, inevitably, a lot to be learned in terms of developing self-directedness from the literature on learning and teaching. This chapter will approach learning and teaching theories from two aspects. First, those related to the planning of teaching sessions to maximise learning and, second, those skills used during a teaching session that will help us develop self-directedness. Throughout the whole chapter we will be taking a transformational approach to learning and teaching. We will consider not only the actual learning experience but also how we will develop learner insight into their learning processes and their attitudes towards learning.

PLANNING TEACHING

Planning is absolutely fundamental to a good teaching session, whether one to one, small groups or large groups. With such a great emphasis on the learner-centred approach it is easy to get nudged away from planning towards a 'turn up and see what they want to know approach'. It is a fine line between belief in learner centredness and an aversion to planning. Planning is of such importance because although in adult learning the objectives are often best determined by the learner, the nature and process of the learning still needs careful consideration.

Learning is new information being placed into the memory in the short term combined with the ability to access this knowledge at a later date. Karpicke and Grimaldi[2] emphasise the importance of successful retrieval (after all, no point putting the knowledge in there if our learner can't find it when it matters). They found that repeated retrieval of the information (not just repeated study) significantly improved long-term retention. These ideas are evident in some of the key models for curriculum planning.

Curriculum planning

> To create a self-directed, self-motivating environment, we need a well-structured programme of learning – the curriculum. A well planned curriculum will help to shape and give guidance to a programme of learning in which practitioners, teacher, assessors, mentor and students become partners in the learning process.[3] [(p. 7)]

Some educators will be responsible for planning and delivering an overall programme of study for learners. This may vary from a very learner-led approach in which the topic for every tutorial is decided by the learner based on their perceived learning needs to a predetermined and fixed curriculum that must be followed. The following models of curriculum design give a flavour of how we might consider the progression of learning whichever approach is taken to topic selection.

Spacing and the spiral curriculum

One of the most well-known curriculum models is the spiral curriculum, which describes a progression that revisits concepts with increasing levels of difficulty.[4] The learner can enter the spiral at the point that is appropriate to their current knowledge and they build upon this as they continue to progress around the spiral and revisit topics at levels of increasing complexity. It is based upon the premise that every concept can be simplified in some meaningful way that allows all levels of learner to access the knowledge.

> One approached knowledge in the spirit of making it accessible to the problem solving learner by modes of thinking that he already possessed or that he could, so to speak, assemble by combining natural ways of thinking that he had not previously combined. One starts somewhere – where the learner *is*. And one starts *whenever* the student arrives to begin his career as a learner. It was in this spirit that I proposed that 'any subject could be taught to any child at any age in some form that is honest'. One matched the problem to the learner's capacities or found some aspect of the problem that could be so matched. That was the spirit behind the dictum.[4] (pp. ix–x)

The spiral curriculum, revisiting a topic over a long period of time, is based upon the concept of 'spacing' which is widely used in education. Research suggests that revisiting a topic at least several weeks after the initial introduction of the idea, called 'spaced learning', is beneficial to long-term recall.[5, 6] It is easy to be put off this idea as educators because when we revisit a topic it is not uncommon to find that learners have no recall. However, be reassured they will reacquire the knowledge much quicker, so don't get too disheartened when you have blank faces staring at you and you begin to wonder if you imagined teaching the topic before. So as well as an overall large spiral to our planned curriculum, there could be repetitive miniature spirals revisiting key topics to help long-term retention of the information.

Interleaving

The ideas of spiralling, spacing and interleaving are very similar to one another, but there are subtle differences and there is also research demonstrating some differences in outcome.[7] As already discussed, the spiral curriculum is based upon the idea of meeting a concept, studying it for a short period of time before moving on to other concepts; the initial concept is then revisited again at a later point. Another consideration in planning teaching schedules is interleaving, which is useful when dealing with a number of similar and/or easily confused concepts. Interleaving involves repeated exposure to the similar concepts in a structured manner, so three concepts a, b, and c that are similar in nature or terminology would be revisited three times: $a_1b_1c_1$ $a_2b_2c_2$ $a_3b_3c_3$. This approach may initially be more confusing for the learner, but long term it improves recall and test performance.[7]

> ### Spacing and interleaving in curriculum planning
>
> When planning teaching in the medium term, consider using spacing and a spiral approach to facilitate improved learning. If there are a number of similar and easily confused concepts consider interleaving them together to aid retrieval of the knowledge. It is important to a learner's sense of achievement that they are able to recall the information when it is needed for real life scenarios or assessments.
>
> *Self-belief, Performance Accomplishments (PA) 8: LT1*

The SOLO approach

The SOLO approach (Structure of the Observed Learning Outcome) also describes an approach to planning learning and assessment with increasing levels of difficulty (*see* Figure 6.1).[8] The learning outcomes are determined first, though they are under constant re-evaluation. The programme of study, the content, teaching strategies and assessment are all planned to fit with the learning outcomes in a process called constructive alignment.

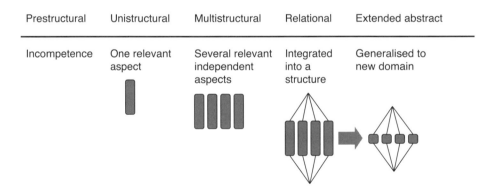

FIGURE 6.1 The SOLO approach to curriculum planning (as proposed by Biggs and Collis)

Scaffolding

Both the spiral approach and the SOLO approach utilise the idea of threshold knowledge – this is the knowledge that is just past the edge of current understanding. In order to acquire this new knowledge and associated skills we need to provide scaffolding (an idea typically associated with Vygotsky's work[9]) so that the learner is given support to achieve the new objectives. Ultimately the scaffolding is removed in a process called fading as the learner takes ownership of the information. There is, however, a suggestion that fading may not actually be necessary for transfer of responsibility;[10] that once the learner has absorbed the knowledge they will simply not use the scaffolding even if it is left in place. Additionally, it may be unnecessary to push for learners to take full responsibility when they are acquiring problem-solving skills. There is a concept known as distributed cognition, which indicates complete fading may not be necessary in most medical scenarios; it is the sharing of cognitive resources so that not all learners need all thinking skills.[11] Distributed cognition is possibly closer to the realities of working life; few of us will work in a completely isolated situation. So with this theory in mind perhaps complete fading of the scaffolding is not necessary or realistic. In the pursuit of self-directedness we should be considering the type of scaffolding we are providing, when we should remove it, how we can best achieve this and how far we need to remove it to represent the reality of our context.

> Because scaffolding is such a dynamic intervention finely tuned to the learner's ongoing progress, the support given by the teacher during scaffolding strongly depends upon the characteristics of the situation like the type of task (e.g. well-structured versus ill-structured) and the responses of the student. Therefore, scaffolding does never look the same in different situations and it is not a technique that can be applied in every situation in the same way.[12] (p. 272)

As is usually the case in education, the specific nature of the application of the theory comes down to the expertise of the educator who must use their own knowledge, experience and common sense to determine the exact requirements.

Scaffolding

Use a supportive, scaffolding approach to teaching new concepts and be systematic and analytical in the removal of this support. Fade the scaffolding to the level that is appropriate to represent the reality of the learner's working environment. As learners develop the ability to perform without the scaffolding, the success will prove motivating as they strive for their own potential in a supported environment.

Motivation, Self-Actualisation (SA) 4: LT2

Competence-based curriculum

There is also a significant amount of discussion regarding competency-based curricula and progression. This approach is of particular importance in the clinical context because there are a large number of skills to be developed as well as the huge foundation of knowledge.

In a report for the US Department of Education[13] the competence-based model (*see* Figure 6.2) is described as the progression to demonstrable competence with a focus on how the learner's traits, knowledge and skills come together to form competencies. The competence-based curriculum expands the curriculum planner's thoughts to a broader approach than simple knowledge transmission or even skill development. This approach to curriculum development combines the skills, abilities and knowledge into a 'learning bundle' that is a context specific competency. These competencies are put into practice and the level at which they are demonstrated can be assessed to determine the level of competence. Voorhees[14] uses the example of a comparison between leadership on a basketball court and leadership in a surgery suite. The competency in both contexts is leadership, but the combination of skills, abilities and knowledge required for each will be different. In a surgical context, knowledge will be absolutely key along with technical skills. On a basketball court the ability to motivate teammates will be significant to the role. There are two different learning bundles put together to make up the leadership competency in two different contexts.

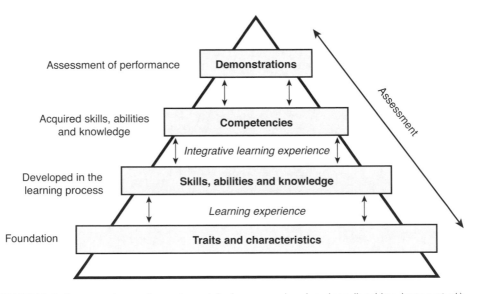

FIGURE 6.2 A competence-based model of progression (as described by Jones *et al.*)

Dreyfus and Dreyfus[15] describe a process of skill acquisition that can be used to determine the level of achievement a learner may have towards a competency. The progression they describe is an interesting backdrop for curriculum planning.

- Stage 1: Novice. At the beginning of the learning process the learner has no understanding of the skill required and will need the educator to dissect and break down the overall skill to allow them to access the learning. The learning will be context free at this point as the learner has no experience on which to base the skill.

- Stage 2: Advanced beginner. The learner begins to recognise how they might deal with the real life situations in which they find themselves; learning becomes more context driven and less about a strict set of rules to adhere to.
- Stage 3: Competence. At this stage the learner is able to cope with the new knowledge and able to apply it in new situations. However, this is done via a complex problem-solving process in which the learner consciously analyses and plans their actions.
- Stage 4: Proficient. After a period of practice and experiencing the skill in a variety of contexts, the learner is able to stop consciously analysing how to approach the problem. They have now experienced enough that they are quickly able to identify the way forward without conscious thought.
- Stage 5: Expert. Finally the learner reaches a point where their approach is guided by intuition. Many educators will be at this stage in their own skillset and as such they must be aware of the need to dissect their own actions in a conscious manner that they have probably not attempted for a while.

Competences

Consider your planned content as a series of bundles of knowledge and skills that come together to form the competence you are teaching. It will be helpful to learners to understand how their learning can be pulled together in this way, especially if the competences can be related to their work requirements. Their progress towards these competencies can be clearly identified.

Skills, Concrete Experience (CE) 7: LT3

The SPICES model

The SPICES model was developed specifically for healthcare contexts and it encourages wider consideration of the whole programme.[16] Rather than describing the path taken by the learner as they progress through the course the focus is on the overall intentions of the programme. The SPICES model describes six axes along which a curriculum could lie; there is not a right or wrong end, rather it is a mechanism for self-audit and discussion about the nature of the programme being developed.

S   Student centred vs Teacher centred

P   Problem based vs Information gathering

I   Integrated vs Discipline based

C   Community based vs Hospital based

E   Elective vs Uniform/standard
S   Systematic vs Apprenticeship

Harden[16] also discusses the wider issue of the 'hidden curriculum'. The combination of the curriculum that is planned and the curriculum that is taught will add up to the curriculum that is learned. Despite everyone's best efforts, they do not necessarily all align with each other (*see* Figure 6.3).

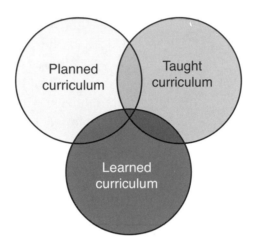

FIGURE 6.3 Aligning the planned, taught and learned curriculum (as described by Harden)

Planning a curriculum is a highly skilled task and one that requires the educator to consider exactly what the learners will learn and how this will happen most effectively. Assuming that the development of self-directedness is one of the aims of the programme, we need to keep this in mind throughout the planning process, not as a bolt-on component. Discuss where on Harden's axis the course needs to lie if the learner is going to take some control. Keep the learner informed about the curriculum structure so they have an understanding of the direction of their learning.

The hidden curriculum

Be aware that the curriculum you plan to teach, the curriculum you actually teach and the curriculum that is learned may not be congruent with each other. Work towards alignment through careful planning, feedback and evaluation to ensure the learning experiences you offer are transparent and structured from all perspectives.

Skills, Concrete Experience (CE) 8: LT4

Without a working understanding of the structure a spiral curriculum can be frustratingly repetitive to a learner while the SOLO approach could seem fragmented and disconnected at the beginning. Ultimately, we have to make sure that what we plan to teach, what we actually teach and what is learned are congruent with one another.

Formative assessment

A significant part of planning for longer term educational relationships involves formative assessment. This is the discussion about the learning that takes place; the conversations that give both the learner and educator a better understanding of what has been learnt and what the next step is. We will not be discussing summative assessment, not because it is unimportant, but because the structure and composition of summative assessments lies outside the control of most medical educators. In fact there is plenty of research that shows summative assessment is important for the learning process as well as for checking understanding because it requires repeated retrieval of the information that helps to embed the learning.[17]

Formative assessment has been in development for many years now and has become increasingly important in education. In the 1990s the government was well on the way to producing the school education system we know today – a National Curriculum, GCSEs, League tables, but policy was primarily based upon research into direct relationships between inputs into the classroom and outcomes from the classroom. For example, how does the experience of the teacher affect the grades of the lowest achieving pupils? How does the length of the lesson affect the levels of satisfaction among staff and students? Research questions such as these did not address what was actually happening in the classroom. However, there was an increasing pool of research on formative assessment and in 1998 Black and Wiliam[18] published a review of this research covering 250 articles and chapters across a range of contexts. They entitled it *Inside the Black Box*, where the black box represents the classroom and they drew together a number of aspects of formative assessment in the classroom that had been found to improve outcomes.

These ideas have become the basis for Assessment for Learning; a concept (almost) fully embedded within primary and secondary education across the country. This has been, at least in part, a consequence of the Assessment for Learning Strategy.[19] In fact, many of the ideas have also found their way into adult education and, in particular, medical education. However, the overall concept has not made the transition as successfully.[20]

In the original research by Black and Wiliam[18] there was no mention of the phrase Assessment for Learning; they talked about formative assessment and in reality the term formative assessment is often used interchangeably with 'Assessment for Learning'. However, we need a pinch of caution because the common usage of the term formative assessment is to describe the discussion and/or feedback after a learner receives a summative grade. Assessment for Learning certainly includes this dialogue, but its impact spreads much further. For a successful dialogue about learning the educator has to make sure that the learner can talk about their learning. Definitions of Assessment for Learning are plentiful and I would suggest that the actual terminology used (formative assessment or Assessment for Learning) does not really matter at the frontline. As long the general principle is understood and taken on board you could call it a chocolate teapot if you like. The original definition of this broad approach to formative assessment was suggested by Black and Wiliam.

> All those activities undertaken by teachers, and by their students in assessing them-selves, which provide information to be used as feedback to modify the teaching and learning activities in which they are engaged. Such assessment becomes 'forma-tive assessment' when the evidence is actually used to adapt the teaching work to meet the needs.[18] (p. 2)

An alternative definition came from Looney:

> Formative assessment refers to the frequent, interactive assessments of student progress to identify learning needs and shape teaching.[21] (p. 5)

Where Looney says frequent, Stiggins[22] says 'continuous' which demonstrates how deeply these principles need to be embedded in everything that an educator does. Assessment for Learning is not just specific activities or checkpoints planned into the programme.

So the central idea is that the teacher will gain information about the learning taking place, which should be used to guide future planning. This is done quite instinctively by many – when we notice that our learner really hasn't got to grips with a topic we will probably revisit it in another way at some point in the future. We can take it a step further by actually planning how we will gain information about the learner's understanding rather than simply 'noticing'. We can also plan how we will ensure that the learner has the knowledge, skills and opportunity to discuss and demonstrate their learning adequately. Otherwise the information used to guide future planning is at best incomplete and potentially totally inaccurate. For this to be the case the learner needs to know what they are learning; they should be able to recognise when they have achieved it and understand how well they have achieved. So educators need to provide the learner with information about their learning alongside the tools and opportunities for the learner to tell the educator about what they have learned. This is seen to be achieved through four main aspects of teaching:

sharing success criteria (learning objectives and learning outcomes); questioning; modelling, peer assessment and self-assessment; and feedback. The specifics of each aspect will be looked at in more detail in the following section on the teaching session. Here we are only considering the impact of the general principle of Assessment for Learning on short, medium and long-term planning.

Essentially, Assessment for Learning is a dialogue about learning between the educator and learner and is fundamentally linked with self-directedness. It is providing the learner with an understanding of their learning that is fundamental to their ability to navigate the learning cycle by themselves.

> Efforts to build self-regulation and autonomy begin with learners' partnership in the assessment and learning process. The fundamental objective of the theory of formative assessment is to equip students with self-regulated learning strategies which sustain stable motivation.[23 (p. 241)]

Assessment for Learning

Use the principles of Assessment for Learning to ensure learners are part of a dialogue about learning. When learners understand what they are learning, what the outcome looks like and their current position in relation to this, they will be better placed to determine the next steps to take to achieve their chosen goal.

Skills, Active Experimentation (AE) 6: LT5

Problem-based learning

Problem-based learning (PBL) rose to prominence in the 1980s when Barrows and Tamblyn[24] began using it in medical education in Canada and it is now being used with success around the world [25-28] and in multiple disciplines.[29, 30] The general principle involves groups of learners solving problems and in doing so identifying and working towards their own group learning objectives. Obviously the idea of using a problem as the basis for learning was not new but the design in the approach to the problem was different and very learner-centred. It is this specific approach that provides learners maximum benefit of a truly problem-solving process.[31] As a learning process it fits well with many learning theories: constructivism, experiential learning and transformational learning are all evident in the process. As a teaching strategy it offers the opportunity to use real examples (even real live patients[32]) to emphasise experiential learning and utilise the strength of emotional memory. In fact, PBL ticks a lot of boxes, but most importantly for us, it is a fundamentally self-directed approach. There will be a tutor taking on the role of facilitator in some way and they may use a heavier or lighter touch depending on group needs. Learners are not learning in isolation but as part of a group, however, the skills that will be built up throughout the PBL process, such as critical thinking which is recognised as a skill fostered through group work,[33] are certainly conducive to a self-directed approach to learning in the future.

> The student-centred nature of PBL, the fact that students start working on a prob-
> lem before they have received other curriculum inputs, the identification of their
> knowledge deficits, the generation of their own learning issues, students' indi-
> vidual study, the critical evaluation of the literature resources, the application of
> the new knowledge to the problem, and the critical and collaborative reflection
> on their self-directed learning skills are all crucial features that foster self-directed
> learning.[34] (p. 415)

The first step to developing a PBL programme is designing a problem. Hung[35] devised the 3C3R approach which gives us three core components and three processing components to consider when producing problems for problem-based learning.
- Content: choose problems that encompass a wide (but not too wide) scope of potential learning and those that will force learners to work hard to uncover the new knowledge.
- Context: keep the problem within a relevant context as this is the most effective way to engage learners and to help learners as they encounter similar issues in the future.
- Connection: use the problem to encourage learners to think 'across' their compartmentalised knowledge.
- Researching: learners must be given problems that provide the opportunity to research within a narrow enough constraint; that is, the combination of content and context provide a sensible-sized region of study.
- Reasoning: learners will need to analyse information, to carry out thought experiments to actively select or deselect options for the solution.
- Reflecting: by providing an opportunity for reflection within the problem-based learning process, the learner has the chance to fully embed the new concepts.

Once the problem has been designed, the process of PBL itself will need to be facilitated. The general process can be described in eight stages:
1. Set the climate
    a. Assign roles
    b. Make/review ground rules
    c. Review thinking and learning processes

2. Read the problem/trigger
   a. Clarify key facts and unknown terms
   b. Contextualise the problem according to the realities of one or more people on the team. Focus on one specific programme
3. Define the kernel of the problem/trigger
   a. Initial ideas
4. Brainstorm
   a. Ideas/explanations
   b. Responses and examples in relations to your experience
5. Discuss and synthesise
   a. Discuss the problem
   b. Summarise what you currently know about key issues
6. Formulate learning issues
   a. Name the key issues that you need to study further and phrase these as questions
7. Independent study
   a. Work on learning issues
   b. Synthesise critically what this learning means for the problem
8. Co-constructing knowledge and professional action
   a. Debate learning issues from literature and practice
   b. Summarise the learning as it relates to the problem and professional practice
   c. Make and carry out an action plan[36]

There have been many advantages of the PBL approach discussed in literature. First, this style of learning encourages the learner to enter their liminal space (sounds a little odd I know but bear with me). The liminal space is that space between the old and new ways of knowing/being/doing, depending on which axis is being considered (*see* Figure 6.4). It helps learners think at the edge of their threshold of knowledge and allows them to take charge of pushing this threshold outwards. When educators take the role of 'imparting wisdom' to learners it is very hard to find this threshold. There is a good chance the knowledge will be already known and therefore well within the threshold, or so completely new that it is too far past the threshold for learners to grasp. PBL allows learners to identify their own threshold and push past it into the liminal space.[37]

In a similar vein, Savin-Baden and Howell Major[38] discuss PBL and how learners will often progress from an initially surface learning approach to the problem to deep then strategic learning.[39]

- Surface learning is a simple rote memory approach. The learner accesses the information at a very low level, unable to see wider contexts or understand generalised examples.

- Deep learning is a more engaged approach. The learner interacts with the learning, relates ideas to previous knowledge and to differing contexts/examples. They will be able to reflect on and critically analyse new information and evidence placed before them.
- Strategic learners are those that are striving to obtain the highest grade possible. They are the ones at school that always had a spare pen or five and always have the right ruler. These learners are very organised and put an extraordinary amount of effort into their learning in order to gain the most from their time as a learner.

PBL will encourage learners to embark upon deeper learning and to take a more strategic approach to their learning as they begin to take control.

There is just time for a quick note of caution with PBL activities. When there is a curriculum and/or an exam, learners often experience anxiety that their learning objectives are not appropriate to guide them towards success. It may therefore be necessary to provide some guidance with learning objective setting to avoid the anxiety becoming prohibitive to learning.[28]

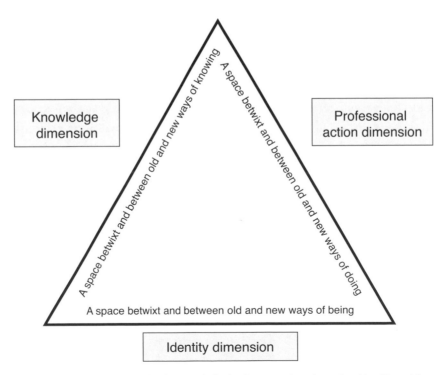

FIGURE 6.4 The axis around the learner's liminal space (as described by Barrett)

> ### A strategic approach
>
> The development of a strategic approach to learning will help learners approach all aspects of their education, including exams, in a more prepared state. An increase in preparedness will help the reduction of anxiety in high-stress situations.
>
> *Self-belief, Emotional Arousal (EA) 7: LT6*

PBL enhances collaborative learning skills that may appear to be at odds with the idea of self-directed learning. However, there is certainly room within our definition of self-directedness for self-directedness towards a common learning goal. Self-directedness need not exclude collaboration; a self-directed person does not have to be selfish in their pursuit of improvement. We did discuss, way back in Chapter 1, that it is possible to be too self-directed. The inclusion of PBL in a programme will ensure that learning skills are honed in a collaborative environment as well as one of individual gains.

PBL techniques are primarily seen as group activities with individuals cooperating and learning from their peers as well as taking responsibility for researching and teaching new areas of knowledge. However, it is possible to take the principles of PBL and use the case or stimulus for an individual. They could identify their individual learning needs in discussion with their educator and prioritise and take responsibility for follow-up before the next session where the discussion could revolve around the new learning gained. Not quite the same process but similar enough that it may be worth considering some PBL stimuli as starter points even for one to one tutorials.

> ### Collaborative learning
>
> Working and learning alongside peers is important for the development of peer groups and relationships that reduce feelings of isolation. Problem-based learning provides the opportunity to learn and achieve together in a positive environment.
>
> *Motivation, Belongingness (B) 4: LT7*

Problem-based learning

Use a problem-based learning approach to teaching that will support learners in achieving their own personal objectives. In this type of learning the learner is able to work at their own pace and at the limits of their own abilities where they can be motivated without being bored or demoralised by too little or too much information.

Motivation, Self-Actualisation (SA) 5: LT8

TEACHING SKILLS

Teaching and learning styles

Learning styles, in the form of VARK[40] preferences and Honey and Mumford's[41] learning preferences, have already been discussed in Chapter 3. The discussions in relation to self-directedness have so far involved the development of learner insight into their own preferences. This will allow them to select and plan future learning opportunities that are most likely to result in success. In this chapter we will consider the need to match the teaching style to the learner while simultaneously encouraging their progression towards self-directedness.

The Staged Self-Directed Learning Model[42] describes four stages of learner and four corresponding stages of teacher that need to be matched for an effective learning environment (*see* Figure 6.5). The model has roots in situational leadership because self-directedness is seen to be at least partly situational in nature.

- **Stage 1** students are **dependent**
  These learners are passive and often need to be led and/or pushed through the learning process. It is not necessarily a bad thing to be a dependent learner; it can be a quick way for the learner to take a lot of information on board. These learners are also not necessarily 'lazy'; they may be very organised and hard-working, but they may be used to a very traditional, 'sage on the stage' style of teaching.
- **Stage 1 teachers are authoritarian**
  To teach a stage 1 learner the educator must set themselves up as a credible expert that is trusted by the learner. With a level of trust in place the educator can begin to hand over small elements of control to the learner.
- **Stage 2** learners are **interested**
  Stage 2 learners are or can be motivated learners. They will engage willingly with the content of the learning and have some understanding of the learning process.
- **Stage 2 teachers are motivators or guides**
  To teach a stage 2 learner the educator must be enthusiastic enough to get these

learners onside and provide a sound rationale of the need to learn the content. This will provide a foundation from which learners can pursue further learning for themselves.

- **Stage 3** learners are **involved**

  These learners consider themselves to be part of the learning process, not simply learners in a content-driven, teacher-led experience. Stage 3 learners do not have the teacher placed upon a pedestal, as they will believe that they could at some point become an equal to the teacher.

- **Stage 3 teachers are facilitators**

  To teach stage 3 learners the teacher becomes a facilitator; they share learning decisions and engage in (almost) equal conversations with the learner. Learners at this stage will work well in small, independent groups who have been assigned specific tasks.

- **Stage 4** learners are **self-directed**

  The stage 4 learner is the learner that will meet our definition of self-directed; they will seek out their own learning opportunities. They have self-insight and an understanding of the learning process and resources available to them that allows them to successfully pursue their chosen learning objectives.

- **Stage 4 teachers are consultants or delegators**
- Teaching stage 4 learners will involve delegating the learning to the learner and mentoring them through the process. The degree and type of involvement will vary from learner to learner, but the teacher must be aware of the need to remain

	T1 teacher Authoritarian	T2 teacher Motivator	T3 teacher Facilitator	T4 teacher Delegator
S4 learner Self-directed	Severe mismatch	Mismatch	Near match	Match
S3 learner Involved	Mismatch	Near match	Match	Near match
S2 learner Interested	Near match	Match	Near match	Mismatch
S1 learner Dependent	Match	Near match	Mismatch	Severe mismatch

FIGURE 6.5 Grow's Staged Self-Directed Learning model

in the backseat for these learners. They are often so engaged that it is enjoyable to participate in learning conversations with stage 4 learners, but it is easy to become overly involved. This will probably not aid their self-directedness and may even be frustrating for them as they will want to be in charge.

While we are aiming to develop a self-directed learner, we need to be wary of launching straight into a 'delegator' approach that could prove to be a severe mismatch for our learners. Therefore, we should carefully judge the stage that our learner has reached (keeping in mind that this may vary from task to task) and match our teaching to their needs. Then gently encourage the learner up through the stages towards a self-directed approach matching our style of teaching as they progress. This approach will help them develop towards their potential in terms of self-directedness.

Teaching style

Learners should have insight into their own preferences with regard to teaching style, learning style and self-directedness. An awareness of their natural preference and how this will impact on their ability to learn will help them understand their own self-directedness and successfully fulfil their potential after formal studies by seeking appropriate learning experiences.

Motivation, Self-Actualisation (SA) 6: LT9

Assessment for Learning

Assessment for Learning has already been touched upon as a general principle when planning a learning encounter. Just to remind ourselves, Wiliam provided the following definition:[43]

> An assessment functions formatively to the extent that the evidence about student achievement is elicited, interpreted and used by teachers, learners, or their peers to make decisions about the next steps in instruction that are likely to be better, or better founded, than the decision they would have made in the absence of that evidence.[43 (p. 43)]

What is it that makes Assessment for Learning so important? Well, the findings of the research are key to our quest for self-directedness.

At the heart of AfL lies the desire to create genuinely independent learners who can manage their own learning. It invests them with the skills and responsibility they need to make good choices as they negotiate learning challenges.[44 (p. 17)]

This has been found to be achievable through four particular strategies.
- Sharing success criteria (learning objectives and learning outcomes)
- Questioning
- Modelling, peer assessment and self-assessment
- Feedback

The overall effect of using these four tools in a formative manner was summarised as 'making the students' voices louder and making the teachers' hearing better'.[45 (p. 59)] In essence, formative assessment approaches were found to be very effective in improving the ongoing learning conversation between teacher and student. This means the learner will need insight into their own learning, which will be crucial to the development of successful self-directedness.

Sharing success criteria (learning objectives and learning outcomes)

Black *et al.*[45] explain that while learning objectives were initially identified as a separate key aspect to formative assessment they quickly became subsumed into the other sections. Objectives provide a focus for questioning, guidance for the peer and self-assessment and a context for the feedback. Learning objectives and outcomes are essential in more formal learning encounters; however, it is spectacularly unlikely that educators will set learning objectives for a debriefing session or impromptu ward round teaching.

Learning objectives are those two or three statements describing what will be learned in the encounter. Have you ever sat in training that has not provided learning objectives at the beginning? Makes me feel vague about the experience, leaves me wondering what is coming and not fully understanding how it all links together. Now although I tend to live a significant amount of my life in a state of some confusion, I thoroughly dislike feeling like this when I have undertaken a new learning opportunity and I don't think I am alone. For large group teaching the objectives may be determined by the educator so they need to be shared to inform the learner of the target and clarify the aims of the learning experience. With smaller numbers of learners the objectives may have been negotiated in advance so the learner(s) have been part of their development.

The learning outcomes are generally much more specific and indicate exactly what the learner will be able to do if they achieve the objective. So, for example, the objective could be 'to be able to make a banoffee cheesecake' (a personal favourite). The related outcomes would be the learner will be able to construct a base made of chocolate biscuits (a certain oat-based biscuit variety), will know how to slice and cook the banana, will be able to correctly select the ingredients to make the cheese filling and finally will be able to decorate the cheesecake with banana and choco-late flakes. It is a seriously good dessert. These outcomes make it very clear to the learner what they will be able to do when they achieve the objective, they will be able to deconstruct their own learning. Perhaps they are not yet able to get the mix of biscuit and honey right for the base but the rest came out great, they know exactly what to improve next time without necessarily needing feedback because the learn-ing requirements have been made so clear to them.

Many adult learning encounters in medical education are learner led (such as problem-based learning already discussed) where the learning objectives are decided by the learner. Sometimes this is in advance of teaching so the educator can prepare suitable learning experiences. Where this is the case it is helpful for the learner if the educator constructs learning outcomes related to the objectives provided.

While learning objectives and outcomes are always useful it is important to avoid them becoming constraining factors for learning. Learners may have 'burning issues' to deal with or specific patient encounters that are an excellent source of experien-tial learning and there is certainly value in discussing them. As long as the learning remains relevant (where to buy the best coffee is not on the curriculum) a degree of flexibility may be sensible, even if it means not meeting the learning outcomes by the end of the session – these can be incorporated another time.

Objectives and outcomes

Provide learning objectives and learning outcomes when appropriate to keep the learner informed about what they are learning and how they will know if they have learned it. This will help them develop self-regulatory processes that identify their own further learning needs, sometimes without the need for feedback, and also improve their openness to future learning experiences.

Skills, Concrete Experience (CE) 9: LT10

Questioning

Questioning forms such a substantial part of so many learning encounters in medical education that it fully deserves proper consideration for this model. The questions that you ask are subconsciously telling the learner what they are expected to know and this setting of expectations is important for progression of knowledge and skills and also for self-directedness. There are a number of tools that can be used to help educators improve their questioning, but the most effective and simplest used by

Black *et al.*[45] was 'wait time'. Research[46] had shown a number of positive effects of a longer wait after a question and after a learner response before intervention in the form of either a follow-up question or even the answer. In the medical education arena this is often called 'use of silence', something that many are very skilled at using with patients. Therefore, it is hopefully a relatively straightforward task for many to make sure this skill is also used with learners.

Probably the most well-known classification of questions is 'open/closed', which has already been touched upon in Chapter 4. Closed questions will close down the conversation; they usually require little thought from the learner, whereas open questions will be more expansive. An alternative way to classify questions in a similar vein is 'productive/reproductive'.[47] A reproductive question requires the learner to reproduce prior knowledge, to regurgitate simple understanding whereas a productive question will produce further discussion. Or even 'fat/thin' or 'hot/cold' questions. You get the idea. Whatever works best for you.

We can also categorise questions into levels of challenge. Higher order questions will provide better learning of factual information but also of critical thinking skills.[48] A commonly used tool for analysing questions uses Bloom's Taxonomy.[49] This was a categorisation of six aspects of knowledge that were placed in order from simple to complex and from concrete to abstract. A number of them had subcategories as well, which at first glance appear to provide rather a lot of detail but actually describe a much clearer picture of what each category means in reality.

1. Knowledge …
   a. … of specifics (terminology and specific facts)
   b. … of ways and means of dealing with specifics (conventions, trends and sequences, classifications and categories, criteria, methodology)
   c. … of universals and abstractions in a field (principles and generalisations, theories and structures)
2. Comprehension
   a. Translation
   b. Interpretation
   c. Extrapolation
3. Application
4. Analysis …
   a. … of elements
   b. … of relationships
   c. … of organisational principles
5. Synthesis
   a. Production of a unique communication
   b. Production of a plan or proposed set of operations
   c. Derivation of a set of abstract relations

6. Evaluation
   a. Evaluation in terms of internal evidence
   b. Judgements in terms of external criteria

This provides us with a structure within which to construct questions to elicit high-level thinking from our learners. Low-level thinking questions rely on recall and basic descriptive knowledge that will not encourage our learners to develop the thinking skills necessary for effective independent learning. These six categories were later refined by Krathwohl[50] into four domains:

- factual knowledge
- procedural knowledge
- conceptual knowledge
- metacognitive knowledge.

This is a similar grading system to Bloom's but if, like me, you have a memory like a sieve, you may find it easier to recall four domains than six.

Questioning is clearly important for high-quality learning, but it also forms part of a modelling process that will guide learners in future self-directed learning experiences. The questions that encourage them to think from different perspectives, that challenge their justifications and rationalisations and the questions that lead them through high-level thought processes will all contribute to their ability to do this by themselves.

High-level questioning

Use questions that challenge learners to think critically about experiences and about their own thought processes. Model evaluative and synthesising approaches using questions to scaffold the learner to these new ways of thinking. This will build their ability to critically reflect on their own experiences.

Skills, Reflective Observation (RO) 7: LT11

Modelling, peer assessment and self-assessment

Modelling is sometimes omitted from this section, but its inclusion is important; peer and self-assessment have to be combined with modelling to ensure that the overall process is effective. Research by Black *et al.*[45] identified three key recommendations to help improve the learning process using peer and self-assessment. First, ensure learners fully understand the criteria against which they are being judged. If these criteria are abstract in nature, show them how to complete the task successfully

– modelling. These types of exercises may involve showing the good, the bad and the ugly. Sometimes allowing a learner to see something done badly provokes as useful a discussion as seeing it done perfectly, or even better the comparison between the two can demonstrate the way forward for the learner. The second recommendation was that students need to be taught the skills for peer assessment and self-assessment. We cannot assume that all learners are able to critically analyse the knowledge and skills of others or of themselves. In fact peer assessment is a useful tool towards effective self-assessment – learning to analyse other people before learning to critically appraise oneself. An understanding of the cognitive aspects of learning is crucial (as argued by Brown and Wilson[51]) to the development of appropriate assessment. One of the ways learners will develop this understanding is by seeing the mistakes that others have made and, more importantly, recognising why these mistakes were made. As they develop their insight into the process of understanding itself they gain a better foothold in the overall learning process. Third, successful use of peer and self-assessment requires a close tie-in with learning objectives. Learners should be continually appraising their own learning with respect to these aims. 'They will then be able to guide their own work and to become independent learners.'[45] (p. 53)

There are a number of simple tools used to get learners to reflect on their achievements in a balanced way. De Bono has suggested a useful thinking tool: PMI, Plus, Minus, Interesting.[52] The general idea is to encourage people to scan a problem from different aspects; de Bono is careful to describe the process as one where the individual first scans from a positive perspective, then from a negative perspective, then finally expands their thinking by looking for anything interesting about the situation. It should not be a case of identifying points then deciding which category they 'fit' in. In assessing themselves or others the learner could use PMI to help produce a balanced discussion.

Another suggestion is to help the learner devise their own rubrics for the success (or not) at a particular task; for example, aspects of a successful consultation (*see* Figure 6.6). The learners can develop a number of very specific descriptive criteria, often called word pictures, for each of the three aspects to a consultation (data gathering, clinical management and interpersonal skills). These word pictures describe three levels of achievement: not bad, pretty good and fabulous. In doing this they will be developing a much deeper understanding of the concepts and how they are achieved as well as providing themselves with the tools to critically analyse the performance of themselves or others.

A consultation has to have . . .	Not bad	Pretty good	Fabulous
Data gathering			
Clinical management			
Interpersonal skills			

FIGURE 6.6 Developing success criteria for a consultation (adapted from Smith)

There are many opportunities in medical education for debriefing sessions and these are often focused on the new information uncovered in the previous clinic or surgery. Smith[53] (promoting assessment) suggests that these discussions should also have a focus on how the learner experienced the learning itself: what they found difficult and how they achieved success. This would encourage learners to be part of a continual process of self-assessment and if done in collaboration with other learners they can model to each other the practice of critically appraising oneself.

Critical self-assessment

Build up the learners' ability to critically analyse their own practice through a programme of modelling and peer assessment before guiding them to critical self-assessment.

Skills, Reflective Observation (RO) 8: LT12

Feedback

The final key feature of assessment for learning is feedback.

> Feedback is a key element in formative assessment, and is usually defined in terms of information about how successfully something has been or is being done. Few physical, intellectual or social skills can be acquired satisfactorily simply through being told about them. Most require practice in a supportive environment which incorporates feedback loops.[54 (p. 120)]

Black and Wiliam[18] conducted their research in the classroom so while there is some reference to oral feedback, for most classroom teachers this is not the primary mode of feedback (imagine trying to give individualised feedback to 30 learners). Therefore the focus is on written feedback, but in either case, the general principle remains the same.

> Stated explicitly, therefore, the learner has to (a) possess a concept of the *standard* (or goal, or reference level) being aimed for, (b) compare the *actual* (or current) *level of performance* with the standard, and (c) engage in appropriate *action* which leads to some closure of the gap.[54 (p. 121)]

There is an interesting point to note for those in medical education who do provide written feedback. This is often summative in nature followed up with discussion that would be considered formative, but there is some research in school-based education that suggests this combination of mark and feedback is ineffective (e.g. Page[55] and Butler[56]).

> Interest and performance on both tasks at both levels of school achievement were highest after comments, both when further comments were anticipated and when they were not. Grades and grades plus comments had similar and generally undermining effects on both interest and performance, although high achievers who received grades maintained high interest and convergent thinking when further grades were anticipated.[56 (p. 1)]

It is outside my power to remove the need for summative assessment from those on the front line of medical education. However, we can make sure that it does not impact upon the formative feedback we are providing because it is important for the development of learning skills that learners engage with the formative aspect of feedback. Clearly delineating between summative feedback and formative feedback may make the process more effective.

Formative feedback

Where possible uncouple formative and summative feedback to ensure the learner focuses on the formative advice given and the negotiated targets rather than the numerical value achieved in the assessment. This will help improve the impact of the feedback by improving the chances of the feedback being heard by the learner.

Self-belief, Verbal Persuasion (VP) 5: LT13

Wiliam[43] suggests four possible responses to feedback that will differ depending on whether the feedback is about successful progress or a missed goal (*see* Table 6.1). When we give feedback regarding success we are hoping to increase the learner's aspirations. When the feedback relates to a missed goal we generally want learners to increase, or at least redirect, their level of effort.

TABLE 6.1 Responses to different types of feedback[43]

Response types	Feedback indicates performance exceeds goal	Feedback indicates performance falls short of goal
Change behaviour	Exert less effort	*Increase effort*
Change goal	*Increase aspiration*	Reduce aspiration
Abandon goal	Decide goal is too easy	Decide goal is too hard
Reject feedback	Ignore feedback	Ignore feedback

The effectiveness of the feedback will be dependent on the levels of support and challenge provided. Getting the combination of support and challenge correct will be unique to each feedback context, get it wrong and the outcome will probably be negative. The challenge–support grid[57] (*see* Figure 6.7) describes the nature of a relationship when the different combinations of support and challenge are taken to extreme. If a learner is provided with little challenge and little support there is no spur for development. This is a collusive relationship where neither educator nor learner feels inclined to improve so the norm (whatever that may be) continues. If the educator increases the level of challenge but continues to offer a low level of support, the learner is likely to feel overburdened by the challenge provided. As a result the learner will withdraw from the relationship and possibly from the whole learning process as they feel unable to achieve the task in front of them. Alternatively

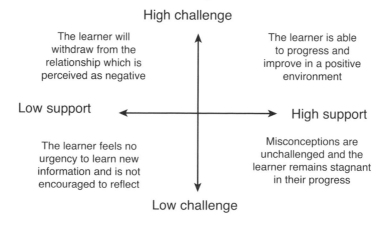

FIGURE 6.7 Daloz's challenge–support grid

the educator may continue to offer a low level of challenge but increase the support. In this instance the learner will have all their own beliefs confirmed. With little to challenge them it is unlikely they will improve in any meaningful way and so will not be able to make progress or achieve in a manner that increases self-efficacy levels. The ideal position is clearly a combination of high challenge and high support. In this situation the learner is able to grow and flourish, achieving in a supportive environment that gives them the confidence to continue to take on new challenges.

By carefully adjusting the amount of support and challenge throughout a learning relationship our learners will be more likely to increase their aspiration or effort. We can build the learner's self-esteem through a process of achievement and encouragement, combined with the ability to accept a missed goal.

Supportive vs challenging feedback

Provide learners with the appropriate amount of support and challenge when giving feedback, take account of the nature of the feedback to elicit a productive response from the learner (increased aspiration or increased effort). A carefully judged combination of encouragement and challenge will help build the learner's self-esteem.

Motivation, Self-Esteem (SE) 4: LT14

More on feedback

Feedback is such a crucial area of medical education that it would be wrong to continue without taking a wider look at research into feedback outside the Assessment for Learning umbrella. Feedback is the mechanism through which the educator

	Known to self	Not known to self
Known to others	Area of free activity	Blind area
Not known to others	Avoided or hidden area	Area of unknown activity

FIGURE 6.8 Johari's window

helps the learner uncover their 'blind' area,[58] that is the area of themselves that is known to others but unknown to themselves (*see* Figure 6.8). Learners with a large blind area are less likely to have successful approaches to self-directedness as they do not recognise their own learning gaps.

Types/levels of feedback

As with much of educational research there is a significant amount of detail in feedback research and it can be difficult to keep it all in mind without using a highly detailed crib sheet. We could look at the eight roles of the tutor in giving written feedback (common reader, editor, reviewer, critic, proof-reader, gate-keeper, anthropologist/linguist/psychologist and therapist[59]) or even go a step further and look at the modern adaptation that now includes nine roles.[60] For one thing these are devised for and are tricky to transfer from written feedback and, second, I certainly would not manage to retain this information. There is an urban myth (or is it based on evidence somewhere?) that the average person can hold seven pieces of information in their minds. I think I come unstuck at five. So I will try to keep it relatively simple and look at a few ways to classify feedback in a manner that helps contextualise your feedback against a background of all types and levels of feedback.

Glover and Brown[61] carried out an analysis of feedback for university level students and identified three categories of feedback.

- Category 1: This is a straightforward acknowledgement of a mistake (but not a correction), such as a '?' next to a written statement or a verbal response of 'nope …'. It can also include simple statements of a personal nature like 'good effort'.
- Category 2: Feedback at this level provides a correction but not any real consideration of why they made the mistake or what changes to their processing may be required. It might include pointing learners to somewhere to find the correct answer, but again it does not really help them process information any differently.
- Category 3: At this level feedback targets how the learner processes the information. They are not only corrected or told where to find the correct information; they are encouraged to think of an alternative solution or a source for the correct information. Glover and Brown suggest that there should probably be an element of feed-forward at this level (something we will look at shortly).

In another attempt to categorise feedback Hattie and Timperley[62] proposed four levels of feedback (still less than five so I should be okay).

- FT – Feedback about the task
- FP – Feedback about the processing of the task
- FR – Feedback about the student's self-regulation
- FS – Feedback about the students themselves

Feedback about the task (FT) is corrective feedback and a lot of feedback is aimed at this level. It can be powerful to provide the correct information on which processing and self-regulation can be built, but it is often very specific to the task in hand and not generalisable. Too much FT risks the learner becoming goal orientated without any real understanding of how to achieve the goal: goals are reached by trial and error rather than through the formation of cognitive processes and hypotheses that lead to 'working it out'. This type of feedback is most effective when it is about misconceptions: where the learner has got the wrong end of the stick. It is less effective when it is simply to point out knowledge gaps. Ideally FT is given immediately as this is the most effective time to embed the new information.

Feedback about the processing of the task (FP) is generally a more powerful approach to feedback, as it includes feedback that helps the learner construct new meaning themselves. It may help them pull together ideas across different contexts, which will enable them to build upon or expand skills and knowledge they have developed in other areas. In some cases it can be effective to combine FP with FT where positive feedback on the task itself will increase the learner's self-efficacy and so lead to greater efforts towards improvement using the information provided about the processing of the task. As a general rule this type of feedback is better given after a short delay in which the learner has the opportunity to reflect on their learning.

Feedback about the student's self-regulation (FR) relates to the feedback that helps the learner improve their ability to self-appraise and self-manage and is inherently important for self-directedness.

> Less effective learners have minimal self-regulation strategies, and they depend much more on external factors (such as the teacher or the task) for feedback.[62] (p. 94)

Providing feedback with regards to how well a learner made automatic adjustments to their behaviours or the insight of their reflection-on-action will help develop those all-important reflective skills in our model of self-directedness. The level of feedback given will probably progress from primarily FT to FP then to FR as we get to know the learner better and are better able to personalise the feedback.

Feedback about the students themselves (FS) is the most personal of the four levels of feedback. Research shows that this is generally pretty ineffective in terms of making behavioural changes. Generalised comments regarding achievement – 'good effort' – have little, if any, impact. More specific feedback about effort towards a particular goal is marginally better – 'you have worked really hard on this project, well done' – but the impact is still minimal in comparison to the effect sizes of other levels of feedback. This is not to say that learners do not like praise; it is certainly important – my one-year-old son gives himself a round of applause and a big 'yay!' when he builds himself a tower if I am not there as his personal cheerleading squad.

There may be a small impact on the learner's level of self-efficacy, although personal praise that is not linked to specific behaviours may be mostly discounted by learners in terms of increased self-belief. It is a fine line to tread between being positive and giving feedback that is discounted. We should try to provide the positive feedback through the other levels by showing them the knowledge and skills they already possess and the successful aspects of their cognitive and reflective processes.

Feedback on processing

Help learners develop a greater understanding of their own cognitive and reflective processes by providing feedback that focuses on the learner's task processing or self-regulatory processes. The learner will begin to understand themselves on a much deeper level as a biological machine with cognitive pathways that determine how they think, learn, reflect and feel.

Motivation, Self-Transcendence (ST) 3: LT15

For our third and final look at types of feedback, we will consider Russell's four types (notice I'm sticking with fewer than five). Many educators in medical education will be familiar with the division of learning and therefore feedback into knowledge, skills and attitude. Russell[63] suggests that there is a fourth important area for feedback that is often forgotten: judgement. This is especially important within healthcare where the right decision could have been made for the wrong reasons or, worse, the wrong decision made for the right reasons. In these circumstances learners must unpick the thought processes that led to the decision in the first place. These judgement-based decisions are key for patient safety so let's look a little more closely at each type of feedback to develop an understanding of feedback on judgements.

- Knowledge – In these cases there is a right or wrong answer and the educator needs to convey the correct information to the learner. If the learner disagrees with the educator, by definition one of them (hopefully the learner) is wrong. Because there is only one way to be right. And the learner has to learn it. Simple.
- Skills – These are practical abilities that will improve with practice. Russell identified three types: physical (e.g. using equipment), mental (e.g. calculations), social (dealing with people, e.g. consulting, running meetings). There will be a range of skill levels and it is important to consider how good the learner actually *needs* to be. Does the learner need to be an expert at it? Or is it something that you have a bee in your bonnet about? I think we all carry around at least a couple of specific things that we believe are fundamental and it can be hard to detach this from the learner's needs.

- Attitude – This is a very scary area to give feedback on and one that should probably be avoided unless the attitude can be considered a professionalism issue. Attitude itself is very difficult to define: intangible and non-specific, it involves all those morals, values, beliefs and prejudices that are based on elusive and vague experiences. It may be impossible to identify the source of a particular attitude as they can be very deeply ingrained. We might like to ignore giving feedback on attitude, but it is sometimes inescapable. When this is the case the best we can do is depersonalise it as much as possible, talk about behaviours as separate to the individual and focus on actual observed evidence rather than vague generalisations.

- Judgements – Finally we will often give feedback on judgements. Judgements are different from skill because they cannot be specifically practised and different from attitude because they are directly observable. The key to feedback on judgements is that we must not judge the learner using hindsight. As we said before they could have made the right decision but got the wrong outcome or vice versa. Additionally, there are often many ways to solve a problem that have equal merit in the given circumstance; this is especially the case in healthcare. Just because the learner chose a different option to you does not necessarily make it the wrong option. The important thing is to discuss their thought processes that led to the decision and together identify any holes in their logic. Look at each of the ingredients (the people involved, the information provided, the background) and help the trainee to develop the ability to respond appropriately if and when a similar situation arises. With judgement situations it is unlikely that an exact copy of the situation would arise again so the aim is to develop their ability to analyse the factors rather than the actual decision.

Feedback on judgements

Learners must feel they are fairly treated by the element of hindsight when receiving feedback on judgements they have made. Focus the feedback on the factors involved and logic they used to come to a judgement rather than the judgement itself to ensure they do not reject the feedback.

Self-belief, Verbal Persuasion (VP) 6: LT16

Types of learner

Russell[63] also described a useful link between learning styles and giving feedback. Activists are by nature people who like 'doing'. They will therefore like feedback that gives them the opportunity to use the new information straightaway. Whenever possible make the feedback short and snappy as they will probably want to get on and try it out rather than sit and listen. By contrast a learner with a reflective preference will want time to think things over, to digest an incident before beginning feedback. They may appreciate thinking time built into the feedback – even if you just pop out to make a cup of tea for you both. Forcing them to put it into practice straightaway is unlikely to go down well. A theorist will like, whenever possible, a theory or model to underpin the feedback. They may ask 'why?' when being given feedback, and this is not intended as a challenge to the educator but an attempt to develop greater understanding of the learning. Finally, a pragmatist will want to focus on 'the what' and 'the how', so feedback should be specific and directly applicable. They will probably want to know exactly what they have to do rather than why they have to do it. All the time remember, of course, that we need to strike the balance between giving feedback effectively and developing the learning skills of our learner.

We can also take into account the level of self-efficacy that our learner holds. Research[64] has shown that learners respond differently to feedback depending on their own perceptions of correctness. So when a learner believes they are correct before feedback is given they will pay little attention to the feedback if it turns out they were right. Any attempt to further challenge them may be lost. However, if they were wrong then this learner, who holds a higher level of self-efficacy, will exert a greater effort to identify where they went wrong and what they need to change to improve. If the learner has a low level of self-efficacy it is likely they will pay little attention to the feedback whether they got it right or wrong, as they are not in the right place to assimilate new information or direction. This is all rather demoralising because it seems there are a lot of circumstances in which the learner pays little attention to the feedback we give. Oh dear. This reinforces how important it is that we work to maintain a high level of self-efficacy in our learners. In a similar vein, high hope of success has been found to indicate a lower chance of avoidance or coping techniques when receiving feedback.[65] So when a learner believes they will be successful they are less likely to be defensive and/or self-defeating in their response to feedback.

Finally, before embarking upon a feedback conversation we should consider the information from the learner's perspective and link it to the competency model of progression. What stage of competence has the learner reached? Do they have a conscious awareness of their weaknesses? The feedback giver will need to consider whether they are helping learners to recognise weaknesses for the first time or unpicking a learned skill so that the learner can add further detail. Often education is about raising the profile of a skill so that the learner can consciously improve before allowing it to sink back into unconscious competence but at a higher level.

- For the unconsciously incompetent learner feedback should be aimed at exposing the learner to the gaps in their knowledge in a sensitive manner while also providing a route forward for their learning.

- For the consciously incompetent learner feedback will need to reinforce the aspects that are positive while providing clear steps for forward progression with easily identified achievement points.
- For the consciously competent learner feedback is about refining the details of their knowledge or skills while avoiding the trap of becoming overly pedantic.
- For the unconsciously competent learner feedback will probably involve gaining insight into the mechanism by which they have learned the new information, unpacking the reflective processes that led them to achieve their goal.

To develop self-directedness in our learners we must help them develop self-awareness of the impact of their learning style on how they like to receive feedback, an understanding of the effect of their own level of confidence and insight into their progression through the levels of competence.

Learner specific feedback

By correctly targeting feedback to the type of the learner, the self-efficacy level of the learner and the insight and competence of the learner, we can maximise the chances of the learner achieving their goals.

Self-belief, Performance Accomplishments (PA) 9: LT17

Amount of feedback

It can be very tricky to judge when we are giving enough feedback. Pfeiffer and Jones[66] described a horseshoe-shaped effect for the amount of feedback. Too little feedback led to collusion between the educator and the learner whereas too much would be insensitive (*see* Figure 6.9).

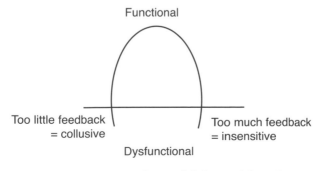

FIGURE 6.9 Amount of feedback (according to Pffeifer and Jones)

Apparently, as educators we need to 'sense' the edge of the learner's comfort zone then push 10%–15% past this. Not an easy task, and we need to find that balance between too much and too little while simultaneously ensuring our feedback pushes our learner just past the threshold that lies at the edge of their knowledge and understanding. Feedback needs to be located right at the edge of the learner's 'zone of proximal development' (ZPD), which is just outside their current knowledge and, as we have previously discussed, the new input needs to be scaffolded into the ZPD through supportive and challenging feedback.

Amount of feedback

Make sure you are providing an appropriate amount of feedback to avoid a collusive or insensitive approach that would result in a dysfunctional relationship. The feedback should be at the edge of the learner's current understanding to push them into new areas of development. By providing feedback and targets at this threshold the learner will take small but achievable risks with their development.

Self-Belief, Performance Accomplishments (PA) 10: LT18

Content of feedback

So, onto the content of the feedback conversation. Where to start. There are so many possible structures, many with clever acronyms, for giving feedback. They are certainly helpful when in the middle of a conversation that has grounded or is circular in nature. They help educators cover all the bases when giving feedback. The most useful model will be specific to the individuals (educator and learner), the nature (level/type) of feedback and to the context. So here we will just take a brief look at a few generic feedback principles.

One of the most well-known is the proverbial 'sandwich' approach. Considered by many as outdated and overused, this places negative feedback in between two positive statements. The problem is that the constructive feedback to help improvement can get lost in the middle with the learner choosing not to hear this bit.

Many medical educators will be familiar with 'Pendleton's'[67] rules of feedback. These have been adapted and altered somewhat over the years and, in some quarters, criticised for being overly formulaic. But in response to this Pendleton *et al.*[67] clarified that these rules were guidelines, not a strict procedure for feedback. When taken in this context the four rules become more flexible and therefore more usable for a wide variety of learners to:

1. briefly clarify matters of fact (but no rhetorical questions)
2. encourage the learner to go first

3. consider what has been done well first
4. make recommendations rather than state weaknesses.

King[68] describes a clear set of six principles for the content of feedback:
1. descriptive of the behaviour rather than the personality
2. specific rather than general
3. sensitive to the need of the received as well as the giver
4. directed towards behaviour that can be changed
5. timely: given as close to the event as possible while taking into account the learner's readiness
6. selective: addressing one or two key issues rather than too many at once.

There are so many decades worth of research and thought gone into the art of feedback but still in 2015 the following view remains the case for many learners:

> Feedback on a task is specific to that task and has no relevance to any other learning. … Such students hold a literal understanding of the term feedback, as backward looking comments on what they have achieved in past assessments.[69] [(p. 115)]

That is just disheartening really. All that effort put into feedback by educators everywhere and yet our learners are still likely to say 'thank you very much' (we hope) and park the information in a dusty drawer in their minds. Sob sob sob. So what can we do? A vital part of becoming self-directed will be in that feedback we are giving and this is why we should stop thinking feedback and think feedforward.[70] Okay, so it doesn't roll off the tongue as nicely but we, and our learners, need to shift our mindsets. Certainly feedback has its place for progression towards specific standards and criteria, but in developing self-directedness we need to provide our learners with information that will help them succeed unaided in the future. Therefore, we need to focus on Hattie and Timperley's[62] FP and FR (feedback about the processing of the task and the student's self-regulation); on Glover and Brown's[61] category 3 feedback and on the skills and judgements our learners are using.[63] These are the aspects that will provide our learners with insight into themselves and how they process and reflect on new information. When learners receive their 'feedforward' they should be encouraged to look past their current experiences and hypothesise about the possible situations in which they may use the new information or insight.

Feedforward

Shift from a mindset of feedback to 'feedforward', guiding learners towards infor-mation and processes that will help them with future problem solving and learning rather than focusing on past experiences. Encourage the learner to hypothesise about potential ways the 'feedforward' may impact upon their future experiences and on unknown challenges.

Motivation, Self-Transcendence (ST) 4: LT19

Receiving feedback

It is perhaps important to consider how we expect our learners to receive feedback. Generally we approach feedback sessions with an assumption that our learners are willing and able to take on board the new information. Whether this new informa-tion is passed from educator to learner directly or derived from the learner through questioning, the learner still has to want and/or need to take it on board.

The idea of a 'criticism cup' is not unique, but Russell[63] suggests that people can be divided into three categories with respect to their ability to take criticism – thimbles, tumblers and buckets. The thimble is only able to take one or two critical comments before becoming openly surprised or even resistant to the new information. If any individual is not expecting feedback they may act as a thimble regardless of their general ability to take on criticism. The tumbler is able to take a few critical com-ments on board before they reach capacity. However, a bucket will seem to have a large capacity for dealing with critical feedback. Buckets usually have a high level of self-esteem and recognise that not knowing is not a failure; it is simply that they are new to a task and they willingly accept feedback as a mechanism to learn. These are genuine buckets, but educators must be aware of those who have a hole in their bucket. These people appear to be able to take on a lot of criticism, but in reality the information passes straight through without any impact. A standard feedback ses-sion with a learner who has a hole in their bucket may begin with the learner stating how terrible the whole thing was; typically negative doomsday type comments. The educator often finds themselves replying instinctively: 'It wasn't that bad …', therefore making it very hard if not impossible to go on to give any actual criticism. The hole in the bucket has 'won' the conversation because the feedback will, at the very least, be extremely softened and the learner has successfully prevented a situation where they have to take on board feedback. Hands up if you have had this conversation.

It is also worth noting the work by Nussbaum and Dweck,[71] which suggests that there is a link between a fixed view of intelligence and a defensive response to feedback. If we can encourage a growable view of intelligence we are more likely to get a remedial approach to feedback where the learner is open to negative feedback and looks at how they can improve. Individuals with a fixed view of intelligence will see negative feedback as an affront to their personal potential.

There are many guidelines for receiving feedback that are all pretty similar in general content. London Deanery[72] suggests the following:

1. Listen to it (rather than prepare your response/defence).
2. Ask for it to be repeated if you did not hear it clearly.
3. Assume it is constructive until proven otherwise; then consider and use those elements that are constructive.
4. Pause and think before responding.
5. Ask for clarification and examples if statements are unclear or unsupported.
6. Accept it positively (for consideration) rather than dismissively (for self-protection).
7. Ask for suggestions of ways you might modify or change your behaviour.
8. Respect and thank the person giving feedback.

Surely everyone working in healthcare will receive feedback in some form or another. Part of being self-directed will be the ability to take this feedback, positive or negative, and to use it constructively to direct future professional growth. If our learners are anxious or stressed when receiving feedback they are unlikely to take it on board successfully, damaging the chances for success and limiting the development of a high level of self-efficacy.

Receiving feedback

Build your learner's ability to receive feedback in a constructive way and support them to take positive and negative feedback without highly anxious or defensive behaviours.

Self-belief, Emotional Arousal (EA) 8: LT20

Seeking feedback

Taking one step further from a positive approach to receiving feedback, we realise that there probably comes a time where we only get feedback when we ask for it. If we ask for it. So when will someone seek feedback? It comes down to a personal evaluation of the cost/benefit ratio.[73, 74] The benefits of the feedback need to be clear to the learner, they have to value the personal or professional gain from the feedback itself otherwise there is little chance they will ask for feedback. However, there is more to it than simply valuing the feedback itself. This value has to outweigh a number of perceived 'costs' to the individual. First, the effort cost involved in actually asking for feedback: will a learner spend hours seeking out the giver of feedback or make repeated attempts if a request gets forgotten? Second, there is a 'face' cost: this is the learner's perception of how others will judge them for seeking the feedback. Is there likely to be a backlash from colleagues if they are seen to seek improvement or perceived favour with an employer? Third, the learner will also, probably subconsciously, consider the 'inference' cost: the implications if they misunderstand the feedback that is given. What will happen if a senior gives feedback that the learner appears not to act upon because they misunderstood it? Put like this it seems surprising that anyone ever asks for feedback.

It is difficult for us as educators to have control over many of these costs as they will relate to the working environment that is specific to the future of our learners. However, we can encourage them to seek feedback in their current environment and therefore build good habits before they move on. This will involve a team-wide cultural acceptance of feedback as an opportunity for all, combined with clear and careful communication at the point of giving feedback.

Seeking feedback

Encourage learners to seek feedback opportunities by providing them with positive and useful feedback experiences emphasising the importance of the process for continual professional development. Through positive feedback experiences our learner can be encouraged to seek feedback in the future.

Motivation, Self-Esteem (SE) 5: LT21

Differentiation

Differentiation is a word that strikes fear into the heart of many teachers mostly because it involves providing personalised learning experiences for up to 30 pupils in a classroom. Fortunately, in medical education, this is a rarer situation, more often it is a one to one or small group context where differentiation or personalisation of the learning is more realistic. It is undeniably important to make adjustments to learners' ability level and also to the level they are expected to achieve. Essentially, this comes back to goal setting and making them realistic but challenging; too difficult or too easy and the learner may become demoralised. However, there is a note of caution (isn't there always?) when you are setting your expectations of your learners. Known as the Pygmalion effect and the Golem effect, our expectations can impact upon the learner's actual achievement. The Pygmalion effect is the increase in achievement by the learner (or employee) when the educator (or manager) has high expectations – a potentially powerful tool. The Golem effect is the opposite, and this is where we need to be careful; if we set our expectations too low we may actually cause our learner to achieve lower than their potential. There is a significant amount of literature about these effects, but it is a tricky area in which to carry out research, simply because the ethics involved in deliberately trying to negatively affect an individual's achievements are rather grey to say the least.

Learners in need of additional support

Learners who find they struggle to meet the requirements of a placement or training scheme are possibly one of the greatest challenges (and biggest fears) for educators. There is no single quick fix for supporting them; in fact many of the skills discussed in this book will help these learners in particular. There is evidence that formative assessment principles are actually at their most effective for lower achieving learners.

> Many of [these studies] show that improved formative assessment helps the (so-called) low attainers more than the rest, and so reduces the spread of attainment whilst also raising it overall.[18] (p. 4)

The coaching skills discussed in Chapter 4 are all key to working with these learners. Often the biggest challenge is developing the learner's insight into their own strengths and weaknesses and encouraging self-awareness. Much of this can be achieved through processes described in Chapter 3.

Diagnostic process applied to learners in need of additional support

When a learner is struggling it is important to make sure the root cause is uncovered before attempting to find a solution. Otherwise, we are going at the problem backwards and trying to find the solution before we have the specific problem. The RDMp model[75] provides a diagnostic tool to identify where in the learner's practice the problem lies.

- Relationships
  - Empathy
  - Communication skills
  - Negotiating skills
  - Leadership skills
  - Advocacy skills
- Diagnostics
  - Information-gathering skills
  - Analytical skills

- ○ Decision-making skills
- ○ Examination and technical skills
- Management
  - ○ Managing particular events (e.g. consultation techniques, managing meetings)
  - ○ Managing comprehensive/ongoing events (e.g. maintaining adequate records, managing a full timetable of work)
  - ○ Managing relationships (e.g. monitoring quality of relationships with patients and staff, utilising prior knowledge of individuals to inform approach to patient care)
  - ○ Managing oneself (both in terms of being able to act upon reflections/feedback and being mentally and physically up to the job)
- Professionalism
  - ○ Respect for others
  - ○ Respect for position (in terms of understanding of their own responsibilities and boundaries and the limits of their own abilities)
  - ○ Respect for protocol

Norfolk and Siriwardena[75] do point out that these are not discrete compartments that will allow each aspect of the role to be easily carved up. As they demonstrate there is significant overlap, however, the analytic process is as useful as the outcome itself. Once the RDMp model has been used to identify the problem another model, SKIPE, can be used to analyse this further.[76] Once again, there will probably not be a single, well-defined factor to take forward to work on. What may become apparent, for example, is that the learner has significant relationship issues due to a lack of empathy and poor management of the situations they find themselves in as a result. The SKIPE model provides a mechanism to explore the causes behind the problem that has been identified in the RDMp process.

S   Skills – Can they do enough?

K   Knowledge – Do they know enough?

I   Internal factors – What attitudes or personality traits may be impacting the situation?

P   Past factors – There could be influences from past events or relationships from any part or time of their life that are part of the causal factors. Be nice, though, because this might be a tricky bit of the conversation.

E   External factors – Look at home and work factors that could be causal in nature.

Once armed with the information provided by the RDMp/SKIPE analysis process you should find yourself and your learner in a really good place to begin making plans for improvement. Of course, the learner must be involved in this process so they have the insight into the analysis.

Diagnosing difficulties

When a learner is struggling to achieve there is a serious risk that they will disengage from the learning process and have only limited involvement in any learning experience offered. Use diagnostic processes to uncover the root cause of the challenges to plan effectively and collaboratively for future learning experiences.

Skills, Concrete Experience (CE) 10: LT22

Learning contracts

As a result of the RDMp/SKIPE process it may be suitable to put in place a learning contract. These are useful for any learner, but they can be particularly effective when a learner needs specific encouragement to engage with the learning process.

Jarvis *et al.*[77] provide the following reason for the popularity of learning contracts:

> Contracts, with their implication of agreement between two parties, seem to provide a mechanism for introducing a measure of order and predictability. All around us the world may be changing; but if I agree to teach you something, this contract between us provides a measure of certainty. What is more, the fact that we have both agreed suggests that we are both happy with the arrangement.'[77 (p. 105)]

The last sentence here seems to be key: 'we are both happy with the arrangement'. The learning contract must not be a one way process in which the educator tells the learner what they need to do and the learner goes along with the process because they will get a cup of coffee more quickly. If the process is done in this manner, many of the advantages identified by Jarvis *et al.*[77] will be lost:

- They provide learners with a greater sense of control over the learning process.
- They strengthen students' motivation to learn.
- They encourage deeper and more holistic (rather than surface) approaches to learning.
- They encourage self-assessment.
- They develop students' skills in planning their own learning, and encourage them to plan for future learning.
- In continuing education, they encourage practitioners to reflect on their current practice.
- They encourage cooperative and sharing approaches to learning.[77 (p. 108)]

So when a learner is disengaging from the learning process, a learning contract in which both the learner and the educator make commitments may prove an effective way to focus everyone's efforts based on rigorous analysis of the problem.

The learning contract

A learning contract can help build a collaborative feel to the learner's progression that works to fulfil the learner's need to build positive relationships. This is especially important where a learner is struggling to meet requirements and may find themselves feeling increasingly isolated.

Motivation, Belongingness (B) 5: LT23

Self-esteem and giving feedback

There are some key issues for trainees who are having difficulties – it is likely they are receiving a lot of critical feedback and this needs to be approached with caution. We have already considered Russell's[63] thimble/tumbler/bucket model for receiving critical feedback. What we did not discuss was what will happen if the vessel overflows. Over time the water in the glass (or thimble or bucket – let's use 'glass' from now on to describe all three, just to make life a little easier) will naturally evaporate and therefore the level will go down. This means that given time the learner will once again be able to take on board additional criticism. We can also reduce the level of water through the use of praise, though the effects are disproportionate – one piece of criticism will need significantly more pieces of praise to counterbalance the effect on water level. However, if we get this balance wrong, the glass will overflow and our criticism will begin to impact upon the learner's self-esteem. Russell suggests three lines of defence at this point. First, the learner will blame the environment: 'The test was unfair', 'It is not like that in real life', 'I wasn't given enough time'. Then, as the learner gets a bit more defensive, they will begin to blame individuals, they go for an 'If I'm going down I'm taking you with me' approach. They are likely to say things like 'But you said I had to …', 'You never told me …', 'The receptionist said …', all in order to shift the blame onto someone else. This is more specific than the vague, general blame shift that occurs at defence level one. Finally, the third defence level is the fight or flight response. It is unlikely (I hope) that the learner will actually choose to punch their educator so the fight is more likely to be a verbal attack (I've seen it). Alternatively, they may burst into floods of tears (seen it) or get their head down and appear to be taking copious notes to make the educator feel they are being taken seriously (seen it). Either way, the flight response is all about stopping the criticism coming.

Defensive responses to feedback

Be sure to take into account the learner's level of self-esteem when giving feedback. A learner in need of additional support will likely be receiving a lot of developmental feedback that may overload their ability to take on criticism. Continual feedback on 'areas for development' will chip away at their self-esteem.

Motivation, Self-Esteem (SE) 6: LT24

Learners in need of additional challenge

In education for gifted pupils there are seen to be two fundamental ways in which they can be challenged – through enrichment or extension. Enrichment is providing learners with opportunities to increase the breadth of their knowledge, setting challenges outside the standard programme of study or curriculum. Extension activities are those challenges that still lie within the 'normal' programme of study but that are accessed at a higher level by the learner. There is an element of overlap between these two concepts; challenges may include projects or problem-solving activities that allow learners to link ideas from different contexts and make more universal-level connections.

Glover and Brown[61] found that higher achievers get less feedback than lower achievers (logical really, fewer mistakes = fewer comments), but is this really right? Here is a question for you: are we targeting a minimum level for our learners or their individual potential? And a follow-up question: do your beliefs and actions match? In the medical education context our concerns for patient safety demand that we focus our attentions to a minimum standard. However, this does not mean we completely forget the potential of our learners so when we get those learners who appear to breeze through, we work to find the additional challenges that will help enrich and extend their learning.

Feedback for high-flying learners

Ensure that high-flying learners are provided with suitably challenging feedback and avoid the temptation to leave them to their own development once they have met a minimum standard.

Motivation, Self-Actualisation (SA) 7: LT25

Educators spend so much time worrying about the trainee in difficulty that, unfortunately, the trainee who appears to be looking after themselves and getting through their exams without causing problems is often forgotten. Books will have an entire chapter devoted to the former learner with barely a mention of the highly capable learner.[78, 79] So what can we do? Well this book is pretty much entirely aimed at developing and supporting these learners. You may have the excellent all-rounder with the skills, motivation and self-belief to achieve potential or a learner who is missing one of these pillars. Either way the strategies laid out in the bricks to build our pillars will support the high-flying learners until they are able to fly by themselves.

SUMMARY

We have looked through a number of areas of research in learning and teaching, beginning with how we might plan programmes that develop a self-directed learner and moving on to the teaching tools we need to nurture self-directedness. What has come through clearly is that the individuality of the learner is the key to success so a learner-centred approach is essential to achieving self-directedness.

In the next chapter we review some of the literature around leadership and management and draw on these ideas to provide the final bricks for our model to develop self-directedness.

CHAPTER 7

Leadership and management

'The most dangerous phrase in the language is, "We've always done it this way".'

attributed to Rear Admiral Grace Hopper

INTRODUCTION

It is significant that much of medical education takes place in the complex workplace of healthcare. Alongside progression towards various assessments and competencies, learners navigate the complex workplace environment consisting of the physical environment, interaction communication, self-awareness, tasks, feeling and learning.[1] It therefore seems reasonable that there may be parallels to be drawn between workplace research and education. This would certainly not be the first time that medical education has learned from research into the business world: we have already mentioned Grow's Staged Self-Directed Learner Model[2] from situational management.

The last couple of decades have seen a shift of focus in medicine: from doctor-centred to patient centred, and there has also been a parallel shift in education: from teacher-centred to learner-centred. The unequal doctor–patient or teacher–learner relationship where one side has a predetermined authority while the other responds as a passive receiver of information or advice has evolved into a joint venture. The consistency and success of this shift in focus is an argument for another day,[3] but it is certain that a patient- or learner-centred approach has been the political and policy level focus for many years now. The healthcare provider and the educator now share a role of facilitator and supporter; they are a provider of learning opportunities. Business has also seen a similar shift in power, from business-centred to customer-centred. The Internet, and more recently social media, has empowered the reviewing and comparing public. This shift of focus in business has been reflected by the rise in the perceived importance of leadership. Management skills have long been recognised as a requirement to make things happen, and leadership skills are now seen as necessary for the broader vision that allows a business to move forwards. The leader has to empower their staff, to encourage self-directed employees and develop distributed leadership using similar skills to the healthcare educator.

There is a significant amount of literature trying to pin down the exact differences between a manager and a leader and more still on the difference between a leader and leadership. These discussions are not of particular significance for our purpose, especially since in the healthcare context one person often has to carry out the role of both manager and leader. Kotter[4] suggests three core roles for the modern manager: planning and budgeting, organising and staffing, controlling and problem solving, which together bring about 'a degree of order and consistency to key dimensions like the quality and profitability of products.'[4 (p. 4)] He suggests a different set of three roles for leaders: establishing direction, aligning people, motivating and inspiring, which combine to produce movement and change.

Current research suggests that leadership is a skill that we can learn through practice. Some will be naturally better at it than others as is the case with any skill. If we can develop leadership skills in our learners we will also be helping them to develop the traits that they need for self-directedness. There is a tendency for us to manage our learners' learning rather than lead it and their level of self-directedness will suffer as a result of this. With strong management and weak leadership, Kotter[4] suggests that an organisation will become rigid and lacking in innovation as there is a strong focus on rules, timeframes and fitting people to organisational needs. Therefore, this chapter will not only consider the development of our learners' leadership skills but also those of educators. At the other extreme Kotter[4] suggests that strong leadership without strong management could lead to an out of control situation with missed deadlines and a lack of discipline in work procedures. There is clearly a line on which we need to balance ourselves to meet the right combination of leadership and management as educators and also in developing leadership and management skills in our learners.

AT AN ORGANISATIONAL LEVEL
Organisational culture
Every organisation, big or small, has a culture. This will be overtly obvious through factors like uniforms, use of titles or first names, a company motto or vision. However, there will also be other less obvious and much more deeply embedded factors that will be demonstrated by the words and actions of staff. This might be oft used phrases: 'what have we got to lose' suggests a very different culture to 'we are

a fourth wave organisation'. The overt and covert nature of culture can be described by three layers.[5]

- Artefacts: These are the outwardly obvious factors, the systems, policies and procedures of the business.
- Spoken beliefs and values: This might include 'mission statements' or business aims. Occasionally they might be less official than this in the form of informally accepted philosophies.
- Underlying assumptions: These are often difficult to identify but will manifest themselves as shared values and behaviours. This represents the accepted beliefs that exist within the business that will be adopted in order to 'fit in' in the team.

All working environments from NHS level down to each individual team will have a culture. These cultures will be inextricably linked upwards and downwards as well as sideways in the form of local relationships and competitiveness. In order to develop self-directed learners we must ensure a belief in self-directedness is fully embedded into our culture at each of the three layers. It will be particularly difficult to assess and alter the deeply buried assumptions that individuals carry with them. Schein states that 'the best way to demystify the concept of culture is first of all to become aware of culture in our own experience, to perceive how something comes to be *shared* and *taken for granted*, and to observe this particularly in new groups that we enter and belong to.'[5 (p. 63)] So if we are to work out the impact of culture and how we might adjust this (if necessary) to incorporate self-directedness we need a deeper understanding of the culture we are working in. The problem is that no two cultures will be the same; they will have arisen over time through group experiences from the very first initial group meetings when the team was formed. In these early stages suggestions and approaches that have allowed the group to move forward will have been gratefully received and therefore positively reinforced. The shared emotional responses will form the basis for assumptions about how the team works.

Group culture is difficult to change because the individuals within the team or organisation will continue to hold those beliefs and assumptions that allow them to continue as a member of the group. This deep-rooted need that we have to be part of the group means that culture can persist through all kinds of internally and externally driven changes. It also means that a new member of the team will not necessarily bring about a culture shift because they may take on the group's values and assumptions in order to fit in, so the culture persists despite new members. This is visible when a new staff member joins but is particularly evident when teenagers move schools – the secondary school classroom is a hothouse of group culture and the importance of belonging is integrally tied to levels of self-esteem resulting in a harsh 'in' or 'out' culture. Although the secondary school classroom is an extreme and still maturing microcosm, we must not underestimate this effect in our own working environments. Ask yourself what is the underlying belief about learner self-directedness in your team? Are you happy that it is supportive of a self-directed approach to learning? For your learner? For all members of staff? If not, this will quickly be picked up on by a new learner who will adapt to fit in with what they perceive to be the underlying beliefs of the team in order to become part of the 'in' group.

Group culture might be difficult to change but it is not impossible. Schein[5] suggests a three-step process that combines Lewin's model of change management with cognitive structures to help us manage a change in culture.

1. Unfreezing or disconfirmation

> If any part of the core cognitive structure is to change in more than minor incremental ways, the system must first experience enough disequilibrium to force a coping process that goes beyond just reinforcing the assumptions that are already in place. Lewin called the creation of such disequilibrium unfreezing, or creating a motivation to change.[5 (p. 320)]

This process is about recognising and unlearning behaviours (not easy) that have become detrimental to the group or the group goals.

Schein sees this as a combination of three processes in itself:

- [the collection of] enough disconfirming data to cause serious discomfort and disequilibrium
- the connection of the disconfirming data to important goals and ideals, causing anxiety and/or guilt and
- enough psychological safety, in the sense of being able to see a possibility of solving the problem and learning something new without loss of identity or integrity.[5 (p. 320)]

Each of these processes is needed to successfully lay the foundations for an acceptable change to organisational culture; none is sufficient on its own to combine to form the motivation. Excuses can deal with an awful lot of disconfirming data. Even when the change required relates to important goals or ideals, the related anxiety or guilt can be repressed. This will happen if the individual does not feel secure that they can accept this knowledge without losing face or having to work against their own morality.

2. Cognitive restructuring

This is the process of internally adapting to new learning, the essence of which 'is usually some cognitive redefinition of some of the core concepts in the assumption set'.[5] [(p. 325)] It is more than simply a behavioural change that can be coerced but will often not persist beyond the change period if the underlying cognitive processes haven't also changed. Having said that, enforcing behavioural changes can be part of this process of cognitive restructuring; sometimes the mind will rationalise enforced changes so they become part of the individual's underlying beliefs. There are another three factors to consider in this process (Schein seems to like collections of three).

- Learning of new concepts – for example, what is actually meant by self-directedness.
- Learning of new meaning to old concepts – for example, incorporating the idea of teamwork and self-directedness.
- Learning new standards of evaluation – evaluating the success of a learner's placement by, for example, their level of insight into their learning preferences or their reflective ability.

Each of these can happen as a result of trial and error learning (this has some negative connotations but every individual and every context is unique) or due to identification of a model that is working elsewhere that can be transcribed.

3. Refreezing

Finally, Lewin's model of change requires that the change be fully embedded to ensure that after the initial enthusiasm and progress there is not wholesale reversion. Schein suggests that while imitation learning may provide quicker results, trial and error learning is actually easier to embed and less likely to revert. With organisational culture we have already mentioned that the shared emotions and positive reinforcement of general acceptance provides the mechanism by which culture develops. It also provides a mechanism by which to embed a change. Provoke those shared emotional responses through congratulatory storytelling, emphasising the successes so far. Positively reinforce the behaviours by publicly recognising everyone who took part and celebrate particular achievements. By doing this you make sure that the shift in culture is evident across the whole organisation or team, not just in a small corner which will not be able to maintain a whole group shift.

Table 7.1 provides a series of mechanisms by which a leader, in our case an educator, may be able to embed a specific culture.

TABLE 7.1 Embedding an organisational culture[5 (p. 246)]

Primary embedding mechanisms	<ul><li>What leaders pay attention to, measure and control on a regular basis</li><li>How leaders react to critical incidents and organisational crises</li><li>How leaders allocate resources</li><li>Deliberate role modelling, teaching and coaching</li><li>How leaders allocate rewards and status</li><li>How leaders recruit, select, promote and excommunicate</li></ul>
Secondary articulation and reinforcement mechanisms	<ul><li>Organisational design and structure</li><li>Organisational systems and procedures</li><li>Rites and rituals of the organisation</li><li>Design of physical space, facades and buildings</li><li>Stories about important events and people</li><li>Formal statements of organisational philosophy, creeds and charters</li></ul>

Organisational culture

Build an organisational culture that accepts and promotes self-directedness in learners that pass through as well as all members of permanent staff. Learners will take these positive cultural assumptions on board and build them into their own cultural experiences. Once internalised, these assumptions about the acceptability of self-directedness will give them the internal freedom to pursue their own interests and openly work towards their own potential.

Motivation, Self-Actualisation (SA) 8: LM1

Learning organisation

The concept of 'learning organisation' is a specific area of organisational culture that has its own research base and even awards like 'Investors in People' that managers like because they can put them on a letterhead. As with any set of organisational values, the strength of a learning organisation is only as robust as the commitment by individuals. The group value is fundamental to the persistence of values over time and the continuance of the values throughout change. However, if individuals are not committed to their own personal development this aspect will not succeed as a permanent part of the organisation value set. The key thing to keep in mind (as you face moans of 'not more CPD?!') is that everyone has something that will motivate them to learn.

> Learning organisations are possible because, deep down, we are all learners. No one has to teach an infant to learn. In fact, no one has to teach an infant anything. They are intrinsically inquisitive, masterful learners who learn to walk, speak, and pretty much run their households all on their own. Learning organisations are possible because not only is it our nature to learn but we love to learn.[6 (p. 4)]

I am very well aware of who runs my household and they are both under three years old. However, if all individuals were as inquisitive (and bossy) as my children, business would come to a grinding halt because everybody would be too busy asking 'but why …?'. Senge[6] identifies the following five disciplines of the learning organisation.

- Systems thinking: 'a conceptual framework, a body of knowledge and tools that has been developed over the past fifty years, to make the full patterns clearer, and to help us see how to change them effectively'.[6 (p. 7)] This relates to the ability of each individual to see themselves as part of but also separate to the overall systems. To be able to see the wood, despite the trees.

- Personal mastery: 'the discipline of continually clarifying and deepening our personal vision, of focusing our energies, of developing patience, and of seeing reality objectively'.[6 (p. 7)] It is, by definition, not possible to force people to develop their own personal mastery. It can, however, be encouraged through a climate where people feel safe to aspire to their own goals, A working environment where there are no recriminations for making challenges to team or organisational assumptions. Senge[6] describes two ways in which this strengthens personal mastery. First, it provides a persistent environment in which individuals feel their growth matters and, second, it will encourage individuals to respond positively and engage with professional development, which is inextricably linked to personal mastery.

- Mental models: 'deeply ingrained assumptions, generalizations, or even pictures or images that influence how we understand the world and how we take action. Very often, we are not consciously aware of our mental models or the effects they have on our behaviour.'[6 (p. 8)] Mental models are those key assumptions we hold and on which we build our thoughts and our behaviours. They may be very general ('the world is fundamentally unfair, get used to it') or more specific ('bosses never really want you to develop because it devalues their position'). These mental models need to be investigated, identified and challenged. Individuals need to recognise times when their observations become generalisations (this links to the cognitive distortions discussed in Chapter 4).

- Shared vision: 'when there is a genuine vision (as opposed to the all-too-familiar 'vision statement'), people excel and learn, not because they are told to, but because they want to'.[6 (p. 9)] A successful learning organisation will also hold a strong and truly shared vision that is more than simply the 'mission statement'.

If teams have a shared goal that they are working towards together there will be greater enthusiasm for the associated learning and an increased chance of high-impact learning. I certainly find it easier to get enthusiastic about learning new ideas and information when there are others involved. This type of team spirit will be infectious and learners joining the team for even a short period of time could catch it. To achieve this, the vision cannot be a top-down directive, it has to be collaborative – built on and combined with personal visions. This means the leader should also be prepared to share their personal vision with others. We should avoid trying to get 'buy in', which implies a sales process; for a truly successful vision we should be asking people to enrol.

- Team leading: 'vital because teams, not individuals, are the fundamental learning unit in modern organizations. This is where "the rubber meets the road"; unless teams can learn, the organization cannot learn.'[6 (p. 10)] Individual learners will find themselves caught up in a positive approach to learning-on-the-job when they find themselves part of team learning. When teams are in the 'flow' the team works naturally and easily, innovation and creativity go hand in hand with an ability to solve complex problems that could not be achieved as individuals. As a consequence, the individual people in this team will be propelled to learn in order to continue driving the team onwards. We find ourselves, once again, linking back to the idea of distributed cognition discussed in Chapter 6.

In an attempt to bring this together, we can consider the learning organisation concept to consist of three key axioms.[7]

1. Leadership has to be distributed throughout an organisation, not concentrated on a few key, high-flying individuals who have the right title. Those who do hold leadership positions should actively develop the leadership skills of others.
2. Individual learning and organisational learning are linked.
3. Leadership is about *shared* visions and linking intrinsic (individual) and extrinsic (organisational) goals.

So, what is the vision for self-directedness within the team? What do you see when you compare individual Personal Development Plans with the department level improvement plan? Where are the key leaders for self-directedness positioned within the team? Considering these three axioms we can begin to analyse how well the team is geared towards the development of self-directedness in learners and also create an empowering learning environment.

> ### Learning organisation
>
> Create a learning environment where all individuals work as part of a learning team, working towards goals that incorporate individual and organisational needs. Empower learners through engagement with the organisational vision and action plan so they feel a responsibility for the goals and the learning required. Learners within this team will be swept along with the natural flow of the team.
>
> *Motivation, Belongingness (B) 6: LM2*

Change management

Having looked at organisational culture, we may find that it needs to be changed, and we touched upon some ideas for how this might be done utilising Lewin's unfreeze-refreeze model. There is much more to be taken from the change management arena because as well as instigating changes to support the self-directed learner it is likely that we are aiming to initiate changes within the individual learner. This is a vast area of research, but the following two models are a useful structure from which to hang our experiences of change. The first is Kotter's[8] eight-stage process, which is perhaps more useful at a team and organisational level, and the second is based upon the bereavement curve and possibly more helpful at an individual level.

Kotter's[8] eight stages of change is a pretty comprehensive description of the pattern of change management.

1. Establish a sense of urgency
2. Create the guiding coalition (the true leaders may not be the people in charge)
3. Develop a vision and strategy
4. Communicate the change vision (with words and actions)
5. Empower employees for broad-based action
6. Generate short-term wins (short-term goals with attached rewards)
7. Consolidate gains and produce more change
8. Anchoring new approaches in the culture

Although a little cumbersome to remember without a crib sheet (for me at least), this clear structure provides a practical mechanism to implement a change in attitude towards learning, learners or self-directedness. For an approach on a more personal level the bereavement curve,[9] which was originally described as a model for those suffering from or working with bereavement, has been widely applied to people's responses to change. Grief is about coping with a loss and a change often leaves people grieving for the former situation. Kübler-Ross[9] described five stages of grief that are now seen regularly on television so they must be fairly common knowledge, and the ease with which the stages have been accepted indicates how readily people identify with them. The five stages through which we may expect people to pass during a change are denial, anger, bargaining, depression and acceptance as they deal with the loss of the status quo. If this seems rather familiar, it may not just be the television factor, as we discussed it in relation to readiness for self-directedness in Chapter 2.

Change responses

Learners need to have insight into their own responses to change to understand that the natural response to change will involve a number of internal processes that may drive anxiety and isolation. This can be avoided by developing a shared understanding that everyone involved will experience similar stages of loss.

Self-belief, Emotional Arousal (EA) 9: LM3

In addition to general structures for change management, there are some useful analytical tools that can help us to better understand the environmental and personal contexts. In force field analysis[10] the current situation is analysed to consider the forces that are driving the change and those that are acting against the change (*see* Figure 7.1). This is based upon analysis of child responses to 'conflict' (jelly or ice lolly for dessert?); as they move through the decision making process they eventually find themselves moving towards a point of equilibrium. In change management we are looking to shift the equilibrium in one direction or another. The discussion to uncover the driving and restraining forces involved in maintaining the equilibrium will likely be illuminating for all involved.

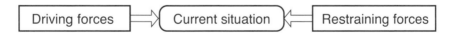

FIGURE 7.1 Lewin's force field analysis

On a more individual level, another analysis technique considers the interplay between survival anxiety and learning anxiety. The former is the anxiety and guilt caused by the urgency for change. Learning anxiety is a combination of three (this is Schein[5] again so it would be three, wouldn't it?) factors: fear of temporary incompetence, fear of punishment for incompetence, and fear of loss of personal identity. So Schein proposes two general principles regarding these anxieties:

1. survival anxiety must be bigger than learning anxiety to allow the individual to move forwards

2. to develop motivation to change we must reduce learning anxiety rather than increasing survival anxiety that would encourage defensive behaviours (denial, scapegoating, bargaining) (*see* Figure 7.2).

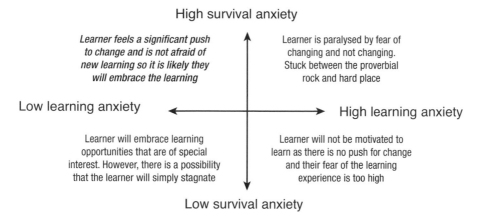

FIGURE 7.2 Learning anxiety vs survival anxiety (adapted from Schein)

Schein[5] identifies eight mechanisms to reduce learning anxiety, much of which is common sense to most modern educators, but having a nice little checklist to help is useful. But then I like lists and I have a lot of them. I should probably have shares in 'Post-it Notes'.

- A compelling positive vision – get acceptance from the learner regarding their self-directedness.
- Formal training: educate the learner regarding the skills they need to develop, and encourage insight into themselves.
- Involvement of the learner.
- Informal training of relevant 'family' groups and teams: provide informal training on self-directedness and its importance to all members of the group to ensure that the cultural shift is entire and that the learner does not feel isolated.
- Practice fields, coaches and feedback: provide the learner with a safe and non-disruptive opportunity to develop their skills for self-directedness. It is probably a poor idea to suddenly introduce the concept as they revise for a big membership exam.
- Positive role models.
- Support groups in which learning problems can be aired and discussed.
- A reward and discipline system and organisational structures.[5 (p. 332) adapted]

Survival anxiety vs learning anxiety

Put in place measures to reduce learning anxiety and ensure you are not unnecessarily increasing the level of survival anxiety. Combining pressure for change without the individual experiencing significant anxiety about the learning will develop a safe but pressured environment for learning. Allow the learner to explore the reason behind their learning anxieties to give them control over similar situations in the future.

Motivation, Safety (S) 4: LM4

Risk management

A significant skill within project management in particular is risk management. This analysis takes place when a change is on the horizon that will mean undertaking a big project of some description. It is also something that we do every day: when we cross the road, get on a plane or decide whether to eat that yoghurt that is a day past the use-by date. So it is very likely that many of us will undertake some form of risk management when we begin new projects or embark upon new adventures, whether that is a new work role or skydiving. The assessment of risk will take into account two factors: the likelihood that the threat will happen and the impact of the threat if it does happen. Combined, these provide the overall risk score. This is sometimes done numerically with each potential threat being assigned values on a scale of 1 to 5; alternatively it is laid out in a grid to visually demonstrate the threats (*see* Figure 7.3).

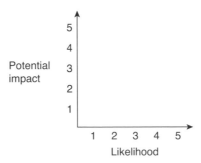

FIGURE 7.3 Likelihood vs impact grid

This analysis of the likelihood and the impact of each potential factor affecting the chosen scenario is a useful mechanism for anyone, learners or educators, to use in assessing a situation. It provides a structure for discussion of hypothetical situations before determining the exact nature of an action plan.

Likelihood vs impact grid

When analysing possible routes forward in learning situations, establish the likelihood and the potential threat of each factor. This will enable learners to critically assess each path and determine the best way forward for their learning.

Skills, Abstract Conceptualisation (AC) 5: LM5

ON AN INDIVIDUAL LEVEL
Being a learner and a manager and a leader
Leadership

There is a significant and growing body of literature that talks about 'everyday leadership'. This is the idea that most (if not all) of us are leaders at some point in our lives and that at times we are leaders without realising it. Even when we are not being a leader we can still contribute to the leadership process.

> Leadership is not restricted to people who hold designated management and traditional leader roles, but in fact is most successful wherever there is a shared responsibility for the success of the organisation, services or care being delivered.[11]

Self-directedness by its very nature involves the learner being a leader. There is a lot (an awful lot) of definitions of leadership – descriptions of leadership as skills-based, traits-based, situational, fixed. The following research by Kouzes and Posner[12] is a very large and widely published piece describing behaviour and characteristics of effective leaders. It allows us to self-assess leadership traits and evaluate the effectiveness of leadership that we identify.

Kouzes and Posner[12] researched the nature of exemplary leadership; they had over two million respondents from around the world utilising a 360-degree assessment tool. They found that those leaders who demonstrated five particular practices were most effective. When leaders are doing their best they:

1. model the way
2. inspire a shared vision
3. challenge the process
4. enable others to act
5. encourage the heart.

They used these five practices to develop 10 commitments of exemplary leaders.

1. a. Clarify values by finding your voice and affirming shared values.
   b. Set the example by aligning actions with shared values.
2. a. Envision the future by imagining exciting and ennobling possibilities.
   b. Enlist others in a common vision by appealing to shared aspirations.
3. a. Search for opportunities by seizing the initiative and looking outward for innovative ways to improve.
   b. Experiment and take risks by constantly generating small wins and learning from experience.
4. a. Foster collaboration by building trust and facilitating relationships.
   b. Strengthen others by increasing self-determination and developing confidence.
5. a. Recognise contributions by showing appreciation for individual excellence.
   b. Celebrate the values and victories by creating a spirit of community.

Kouzes and Posner also identified, through open-ended questions, hundreds of descriptors of exemplary leaders. They grouped synonyms and produced a list of the top 20 characteristics of admired leaders; the top 10 of these are:

- *Honest*
- *Forward-looking*
- *Competent*
- *Inspiring*
- Intelligent
- Broad-minded
- Fair-minded
- Dependable
- Supportive
- Straightforward

Interestingly, this research has been repeated five times (1987, 1995, 2002, 2007, 2012) and each time the same top four have come out significantly higher than the rest. Further to this, three are very closely related to a concept known as 'source credibility'; that is, the believability of the source of communication. Researchers look at three aspects of source credibility: trustworthiness (honest), expertise (competent) and dynamism (inspiring). So these persistent top four characteristics of admired leaders could even be narrowed down to 'credible' and 'forward-looking'.

A discussion with learners considering themselves as a credible and forward-looking individual could be thought provoking. Consider how this may impact upon their ability as a leader now and in the future and what changes they could/should/want to make.

Stogdill's[13] analysis of over 160 studies identified a number of leadership traits. If we skip past the research into common physical traits, social background and intelligence levels, we find a list that appears remarkably similar to what we are looking for in a self-directed learner.

1. Drive for responsibility and task completion
2. Vigour and persistence in pursuit of goals
3. Venturesomeness and originality in problem solving
4. Drive to exercise initiative in social situations
5. Self-confidence and sense of personal identity
6. Willingness to accept consequences of his or her decisions and actions
7. Readiness to absorb interpersonal stress
8. Willingness to tolerate frustration and delay
9. Ability to influence other people's behaviour
10. Capacity to structure social interaction systems to the purpose at hand.[13] (p. 87)

Learners as leaders

Developing leadership skills in your learner will help them develop the ability to lead their own learning. Learners should be looking to take responsibility for their learning, to take risks and persist in striving for their goals. They need to be driven, resilient and focused while also being patient and tolerant of change or delay to give them maximum chance of successfully putting their plans into action.

Skills, Active Experimentation (AE) 7: LM6

In addition to describing the traits and the skills of leadership, there is a lot of research regarding the process of leadership. One of the simplest is that described by Radcliffe: *Future, Engage, Deliver*.[14] It is interesting to note the similarities between these three stages and the top traits described by Kouzes and Posner.[12]

The first of Radcliffe's stages of leadership is 'Future'; the first thing a leader must know is where they want to be – they need to have a clear vision.

> Powerful and effective leaders are guided by the Future they want. And more than this, the leader is strongest when that Future is powerfully connected to what he or she cares about.[14] (p. 9)

The 'Engage' process clearly relates to getting others on board with the move, which may initially appear irrelevant for learners developing self-directedness. However, our learners will be much better supported if they have captivated those around them with their enthusiasm for a particular path of learning. Radcliffe describes six levels of engagement: resistance, apathy, grudging compliance, willing compliance, enrolled, and committed. If a learner is able to engage those around them with their learning goals they will be more likely to achieve those goals.

Finally, Radcliffe introduces the last stage: 'Deliver'. He divides the process of delivery into a series of robust dialogues that a leader will need to have in order to make the delivery happen. Our learners may or may not need to have these conversations with other people, but they may want to consider the importance of having them with themselves. I am not suggesting that we get our learners talking to themselves in the mirror (though that does sometimes work, seriously), but we can help them to use these conversations as markers for their own process of delivery of new learning.

- Making big requests: this could be making requests of other people, such as requesting study leave, teaching or support from family. Or perhaps requests of themselves, such as recognising what they are asking themselves to do or give up to make this happen.
- Maximising the probability of delivery: through ongoing conversations about short-term, stepping-stone targets on the way to the final goal.
- Acknowledge delivery: your learner should make sure they recognise the contributions of others in achieving their learning objective. However, they also need to acknowledge their own achievements. This may mean treating themselves to a beer, a chocolate bar or a trip to the spa, but they should learn to reward themselves because in self-directed learning it is likely they will be their own reward system.
- Non-delivery is addressed: if, however, the goal is not achieved this will need dealing with as well. Depending on the type of learner, it is likely they will either be pretty good or pretty poor at this type of self-recrimination. It is a necessary part of the reflective process (as discussed with black hat thinking in de Bono's hats later in this chapter), but it must be self-managed to produce a positive way forward.
- The wrap-up: the evaluation process in which the learner reflects on the process to identify where they successfully led their own learning and where it fell down.

Radcliffe suggests that we each have three leadership muscles: future muscles, engage muscles, deliver muscles. These need working out and building up, and we can help our learners exercise and bulk up each of their leadership muscle groups. If we can help the learner develop leadership muscles that will help them lead their own learning, we can improve their chances of success when attempting a learning project.

Delivering the outcome

Developing the capability to lead along with insight into the process and their own strengths and weaknesses will increase the learner's chances of a positive outcome.

Self-belief, Performance Accomplishments (PA) 11: LM7

In addition to understanding themselves as leaders of their own learning, learners can also develop insight into their behaviour when working at their best and when they are just surviving.[14] Ask your learner (and yourself) to describe themselves at their best and just surviving; when they are high energy and low energy. Figure 7.4 gives some examples of descriptions.

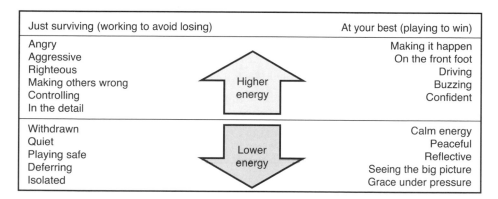

Just surviving (working to avoid losing)		At your best (playing to win)
Angry Aggressive Righteous Making others wrong Controlling In the detail	Higher energy	Making it happen On the front foot Driving Buzzing Confident
Withdrawn Quiet Playing safe Deferring Isolated	Lower energy	Calm energy Peaceful Reflective Seeing the big picture Grace under pressure

FIGURE 7.4 'Just surviving' vs 'at your best' from Radcliffe

Just surviving or at your best?

Develop the learner's insight into their own behaviours when they are 'surviving' and working 'at their best'. There will be differences depending whether these states are reached at high or low energy levels and some learners will indicate preferences for one of these energy states. Recognising themselves as complex entities who behave differently in different contexts involves a broad metacognitive understanding of 'self' that will help them recognise the differences in their own behaviours in the face of success and failure.

Motivation, Self-Transcendence (ST) 5: LM8

Gut instinct

We have already touched upon the relationship between emotional intelligence and self-directedness in Chapter 3; however, it is worth revisiting here as it is an important part of leadership. Goleman *et al.* identified a strong link between high levels of emotional intelligence and excellent leadership.[15] It follows logically from the idea of leadership as the ability to build and convey shared visions, to engage with people and inspire them to work towards a joint goal. Much of this relates to the interpersonal aspects of emotional intelligence. The other side of the emotional intelligence coin involves inward looking characteristics.

Inward looking emotional intelligence in the leadership context brings us to the idea of 'trusting your gut' in decision making. This is the intuition that many successful people say they have about the best way to proceed when there is no strong evidence in either direction. People who don't like the intangible concept of 'trusting your gut' tend to call it 'professional judgement'. In a professional context such as medical education I am not sure that the difference is significant.

In making decisions about the direction of their learning, our learners may have to rely on their instinct to some extent. Once they have identified where they want to be in 5, 10, 20 years' time they can begin to work towards these visions, and some things will be very clear-cut: 'I need this specific qualification to be allowed to do this procedure.' However, sometimes the goal is more vague or requires a generic set of skills that will be developed and demonstrated in different ways for different people. When this is the case, the learner may be able to objectively analyse the situation but often they may simply have to work off a gut feeling that there is a better route forward. So what is this gut feeling? And why do so many CEOs and the like describe times they listened to it with great success and ignored it with negative consequences?[16] Part of the explanation lies in the way our brain processes information without us even realising: 'this helps explain the "aha" sensation you experience when you learn something that you already knew'.[16 (p. 61)] Even when we do not consciously know the information needed to make a decision sometimes our subconscious does because little observations and bits of information have been processed in the back of our minds. Linked to this is our brain's ability to see and form patterns. This means we can take one situation and align it to another, not on the basis of context but as a result of some previously seen pattern we have identified. When the contexts are very disparate this pattern transference becomes known as cross-indexing; this is a highly sophisticated process and one that will become increasingly difficult for the individual to verbalise in a coherent manner. They may not be able to say, 'This is just like when ….' because they have not consciously realised that there is a pattern. To everyone, the individual included, this appears to be action on the basis of gut instinct.

Nobel Laureate and psychology professor Herbert Simon believes that 'intuition and judgement are simply analyses frozen into habit'.[16 (p. 63)] This implies that we need to ensure that our learner will first need to be exposed to analysis techniques, such as cost/benefit analysis, SWOT (Strengths, Weaknesses, Opportunities, Threats) analysis, and PESTLE (Political, Economic, Social, Technological, Legal, Environmental) analysis. As they gain experience in the use of these analysis techniques and are exposed to decision making in the wider context they will develop gut instinct. With time this will help them make the appropriate decisions as they lead their own learning.

Of course the gut is not always right. So the trust anyone has in their own gut instinct comes hand in hand with a need to continually keep check on themselves. There is always a risk that a particular experience may be inappropriately influencing intuitive decision-making processes.

Analysis and gut instinct

Provide learners with opportunities to use different analysis tools (SWOT, PESTLE, cost/benefit) to help them develop an instinct for decision making. These will feed into their 'gut instinct' and give them confidence in their planning and decision making in future learning episodes.

Skills, Abstract Conceptualisation (AC) 6: LM9

Operational capacity

A self-directed learner not only has to lead themselves through their educational development but they must also manage themselves. A significant part of this will be developing the organisational skills necessary to stay on top of the various assessments and get themselves booked on the right courses. There is another important aspect to managing learning and this can be drawn from an area of management known as capacity planning and control: 'providing the capability to satisfy current and future demand'.[17 (p. 297)]

The general idea is that, at an aggregated level, some areas of the organisation will operate at the capacity ceiling while others will have some slack. However, the overall output of the organisation as a whole will be limited by those departments that are at their capacity ceiling; these are the capacity constraint – the rate determining step if you like. If we draw this down to the level of an individual, which department in the organisation of 'you' is operating at your capacity ceiling? Patient time? Paperwork time? Home time? Or how about which of Drucker's[14] four energies are at capacity? Physical? Emotional? Spirit? Intellectual? Don't be overly specific about your life 'departments'; capacity management is also sometimes called aggregate management because it takes a broad, aggregated view that 'does not discriminate between the different products and services that an operation might produce.'[17] (p. 297)

A significant concern for managers is planning and controlling capacity; managers have to plan medium and short term and build a strategy for the organisation. This involves analysis of capacity ceilings and making forecasts of future demands. This process applies just as well to the individual educator or learner (*see* Figure 7.5):

1. identify the capacity ceilings for different areas of life or personality
2. analyse the wider context (a PESTLE analysis may be of use here) to make forecasts of future demands
3. consider how steps 1 and 2 overlap. Is there a high level of future demand predicted for an area already operating at capacity? If so, something needs to change. It may even be possible to put numerical data to each area; these would be entirely personal ratings that are comparatively useless except for the individual and their specific context.

Area of life (department)	Current operational capacity 1–10, where 10 is the ceiling	Predicted factors that might impact upon current operational capacity	Predicted change to current operational capacity	What can I do to increase capacity/reduce current operational capacity, if my predicted operational capacity is above 10?

FIGURE 7.5 Individual operational capacity analysis

By taking this concept far more loosely than originally intended we have an application of an organisational process that provides a really useful way to analyse individual resilience. If we have found that emotional energy is at capacity and likely to be drained by an upcoming exam, stressful strategic meeting or personal loss, we need to find a way to either increase capacity or reduce current demand. This might mean building in downtime that gives more space to deal with a higher emotional burden, or finding a way to deal with or remove the aspects that are currently using up emotional energy.

We need to be careful because 'few forecasts are accurate, and most operations also need to respond to changes in demand which occur over a shorter timescale.'[17] (p. 300) It may be that, even when not quite at emotional capacity, unforeseen events (for there are many) could prove to be too much. Therefore, we need to ensure that in the areas of life where there is less personal control we build in the ability to cope with the potential impact of sudden short-term changes.

Operational capacity

Encourage the learner to analyse their own operational capacity in different areas of their life. Help them to analyse and predict future demands as accurately as possible and identify any potential areas where they will be pushed beyond capacity. The learner will begin to see themselves as an integral part of their context with the potential for two-way impact between different areas of their life and their context.

Motivation, Self-Transcendence (ST) 6: LM10

Being a leader and manager of education

Whether you realise it or not, or like or not, as an educator you are taking on a leading role and with assessments and tutorials there is a good chance you are also a manager of education. If you are getting it right (which I am sure you are) your learners will see you as an organised and effective individual, someone to follow and emulate, and you will have influence over them. This is great, as long as we are careful how we use this power … evil laugh, mwa ha ha. Ahem. Sorry. Raven and French identified five bases of power.[18]

- Referent power: this is strong when the learner really likes their educator.
- Expert power: this is strong when the learner holds the expertise and competence of the educator in high esteem.
- Legitimate power: this is strong when the educator actually holds formal authority over the learner.
- Reward power: this is strong when the educator has the ability to convey rewards.
- Coercive power: this is strong when the educator has the ability to reprimand or punish.

At any particular point in the relationship between yourself and your learner you may find some power bases are stronger than others. For example, when carrying out assessments we hold significant legitimate power, but during tutorial teaching it is more likely that the power base is expert. You may want to consider which power bases are stronger when you are working with a manager hat on or with a leader hat on. An awareness of which power base is strongest will affect how best to motivate and inspire learners. Knowing the basis for power at any one time can help us to make our comments more relevant to the current relationship and so increase the impact they have on learners.

Power bases

Be aware which power base the learner is sensing at different times in the relationship: referent, expert, legitimate, reward or coercive. A learner who feels the power base is coercive may be less likely to respond positively and believe the validity of the educator's comments. Conversely, power based on respect for expertise or based on a genuine connection with the educator is more likely to provide a positive foundation.

Self-belief, Verbal Persuasion (VP) 7: LM11

Motivation

The location of our power base is inextricably linked with the power we have to motivate. Motivation forms one of the three pillars that are necessary for self-directed learning and we have already utilised Maslow's hierarchy of needs as our structure to identify potential areas for action. There are many different interpretations and structures, but since medical education is often in the workplace it is useful to consider Herzberg's division of influencing factors into motivating and what he calls hygiene factors (that is, those factors working against motivation) (*see* Figure 7.6).[19] The model was developed from workplace-based research so it is particularly relevant for the vocational nature of much of medical education.

Top hygiene factors that lead to dissatisfaction	Top motivational factors that lead to satisfaction
Company policy Supervision Relationship with boss Work conditions Salary Relationship with peers Security	Achievement Recognition Work itself Responsibility Advancement Growth

FIGURE 7.6 Herzberg's motivational theory

These factors are not to be considered as opposites; there is not a diametrically opposite factor for each hygiene factor that will be motivational. They are factors that by their presence will cause one or the other, but in their absence they will be not cause the opposite. Therefore, as educators trying to create a motivational environment we should seek to remove the hygiene factors and promote the motivational factors.

Herzberg's model of motivation is based on factors identified by workers about motivational and non-motivational situations. An alternative approach to motivation is to consider the psychological processes behind motivation; whether we cognitively deal with situations helplessly or masterfully.[20] This is closely linked to the concepts of fixed and growable intelligence discussed in Chapter 3. Although this research was actually carried out with children, it is easily identified in adults and research with adults has also demonstrated these characteristics.

The helpless approach is a maladaptive process. People with this approach avoid challenge and quickly give up when obstacles are placed in the way of a goal. When confronted with challenge it is likely that they will provide excuses due to their lack of ability in some way, and they will also appear to get quickly bored with or distracted from the work. They may demonstrate dislike for the task itself or become anxious about their performance.

> Helpless children viewed their difficulties as failures, as indicative of low ability and as insurmountable. They appeared to view further effort as futile and perhaps, as their defensive manoeuvres suggest, as further documentation of their inadequate ability.[20 (p. 258)]

Learners with the helpless approach are likely to set themselves performance-orientated goals with the aim to gain a favourable judgement and avoid showing any inadequacies.

The masterful approach is adaptive; these individuals will not only continue to work towards goals despite challenges, they will actively seek out challenges. They perceive any challenges as obstacles to be overcome with effort. They may be the sort of person who you hear muttering to themselves: 'Concentrate' or 'Come on, you know this' or 'Nearly got it'. While admittedly this does sometimes sound a little odd, it is demonstrative of their fundamental belief that they can do it. These learners will set themselves learning goals with the aim to increase their knowledge and/or skills and they will believe that the control over achievement (or not) lies with them.

Dweck found that when faced with repeated failures, the problem-solving skills of those with a helpless mindset dropped off whereas those with a masterful mindset actually taught themselves new approaches to forming and testing a hypothesis. However, they did also find that even with a fixed view of intelligence, the learner could still approach problems in a masterful manner if they held a high enough opinion of their own ability (*see* Table 7.2). This reiterates the importance of a high level of self-efficacy in problem solving and dealing with challenge.

TABLE 7.2 A fixed or growable belief in intelligence and the outcome behaviour patterns[20] (p. 259)

Theory of intelligence	Goal orientation	Perceived present ability	Behaviour pattern
Entity (Fixed)	Performance – Proving their ability (to gain positive judgements/avoid negative ones)	High	Mastery-orientated
		Low	Helpless-orientated
Incremental (growable)	Learning – Improving their ability (to increase knowledge and/or skills)	High or low	Mastery-orientated

Even though this research is not directly from the world of leadership and management, the implications for motivation are clear and relevant. Learners who demonstrate a growable belief of intelligence (who set learning goals and thrive on challenge) are likely to be intrinsically motivated. These learners find the accomplishment of the task reward enough and research shows that intrinsically motivated individuals tend to achieve more highly, put in more effort, persist for longer, seek out more challenge and are more likely to be lifelong learners.[21] Those who demonstrate a fixed belief in intelligence (who set performance goals and appear averse to challenge) will more likely need extrinsic rewards. This is a key piece of information for the educator, but for lifelong learning it is important that learners have insight into their own preferences. If they are generally motivated by factors with an external locus the learner will need to find ways to make this work for them. Research repeatedly indicates, to the point that it is now seen as core to adult learning (e.g. Goldman[22]), that intrinsic motivation is a requirement for self-directedness. Certainly this is the case up to a point; however, even though I am intrinsically motivated in the main I sometimes need extrinsic motivators: 'When I've finished this question/this section/this report I can have a biscuit.' Unfortunately, this approach combined with the writing of this book has led to a significant biscuit shortage in my home town.

Ask your learner when they feel clever (that may seem like a rather strange question so best put it context, if you ask it as you pass in the corridor you may find they start avoiding you). Those with a fixed view of intelligence will likely answer something like 'when I get a good mark in exams' or 'when I get praise for an answer from the big boss'. The responses from those with a growable mindset will more likely be 'when I am working hard' or 'when I suddenly realise how two unrelated factors are linked together'. Their response gives an insight into their cognitive processing of challenge, achievement and motivation. This, in turn, provides information about how they might be successfully motivated.

> ### Intrinsic or extrinsic motivation
>
> Consider the locus of motivation for your learner – intrinsic or extrinsic. If you can develop the learner's personal mastery you can raise their self-esteem and develop an ability to be motivated by the learning process itself rather than being fearful of failure as measured against some performance criteria.
>
> *Motivation, Self-Esteem (SE) 7: LM12*

Leadership experiences

We have so far considered what the educator can do to develop insight into their power base and the forms of motivation they can provide. There are also a number of more tangible things that educators can do to develop the leadership skills of their learners. There is plenty of leadership in healthcare, not all of it good (insert your own example here), and our learners can develop their own leadership skills by being given opportunities to observe, collaborate and lead within a safe environment. Kotter identified three factors that would promote leadership skills and a further three that would inhibit development of leadership.[4]

Career experiences that promote leadership:

- Challenging assignments early in a career: Stretches people, helping that to grow in many dimensions, some of which will be relevant to leadership; allows individuals to try leadership and learn from the successes and failures.
- Visible leadership role models who are very good or very bad: Extreme examples, both good and bad, are easy to learn from because the lessons are very clear.
- Assignments which broaden: Breadth of knowledge is particularly important for direction setting and breadth of contacts and relationships for alignment and motivation.[4 (p. 154)]

Career experiences that inhibit leadership:

- A long series of narrow and tactical jobs: Makes one short-term and tactically orientated; does not develop long-term and strategic skills
- Rapid promotions: Does not help people to think long term or to learn the impact of their actions over the long term; can encourage a manipulative style
- Measurement and rewards based on short-term results only: Encourage people to pay attention to the management aspects of their jobs and ignore the leadership aspects; teaches management but not leadership.[4 (p. 154)]

There are some aspects of medical education where providing these things will prove tricky, for example, short, snappy rotations that give little time for long-term thinking. However, things like the audits you ask learners to complete will convey underlying messages about the need for challenge and breadth of knowledge. In addition, intentionally or not, you and your colleagues will be continually modelling leadership. For many learners this will be the main leadership message during their training as they will not truly benefit from opportunities to lead until they take up their chosen post.

Modelling leadership

Provide the opportunity for the learner to see others as leaders and devote time to unpicking exactly how leadership has been demonstrated. This is especially relevant where it is difficult to directly provide learners the opportunity to lead or develop leadership skills.

Self-belief, Vicarious Experience (VE) 5: LM13

Managing meetings

Many of us have diaries packed full with meetings and in my experience meetings inevitably add to my 'to do' list but sometimes I actually don't mind. This is usually dependent on whether the meeting was positive, organised and dynamic or one-way information dissemination with some notion of 'consultation'.

> Meetings can form useful ways of enhancing team spirit and solving difficulties creatively. They can also often waste time, increase inter-colleague hostility and paper over deep divisions between points of view.[7] (pp. 166–7)

Managing meetings is a skill and certainly one that it would be useful for learners to develop. The coordination of people, resources and time in a positive and organised manner clearly describes a useful skill set for learners looking to pull these things together towards their chosen learning goal. There is one particular approach to meetings that is of interest for the development of self-directedness: de Bono's thinking hats.[23] Devised and written to help managers run brainstorming meetings, the idea is also easily adapted to the reflective process. The six thinking hats are a mechanism to encourage structured and parallel thinking. Many of us would approach a problem by thinking about multiple aspects at once; de Bono's hats mean that a single problem is considered from a number of parallel directions and not all at the same time.

Confusion is the biggest enemy of good thinking. We try to do too many things at the same time. We look for information. We are affected by feelings. We seek new ideas and options. We have to be cautious. We want to find benefits. Those are a lot of things that need doing. Juggling six balls at the same time is rather difficult. Tossing up one ball at a time is much easier.[23 (p. 11)]

De Bono described six modes of thought with each assigned a coloured hat. When a specific hat is worn all thinking must be in accordance with the allocated mode. Any train of thought that is heading in the wrong direction should be stopped and only continued when the appropriate hat is worn.

- The white hat is a neutral, informational, objective thinking mode that elicits only the facts regarding the situation.
  - In this thinking mode a reflector removes emotion and simply describes the experience; it may help to make a timeline of events.
- The red hat is the 'feelings' thinking mode. This is the opportunity to further develop intuition and gut instinct.
  - When reflecting with the red hat on, consider the feelings of everyone involved to help gain alternative perspectives on the situation.
- The black hat is the pessimistic thinking mode. Although some might consider this a negative impact upon a discussion, reflective or otherwise, in reality often some caution is needed and a true evaluative process needs to consider what went wrong.
  - This is a logical and specific mode, not an emotional one, so keep evaluative comments based in fact and consider if, how and why things went wrong, and whether there were any points that exacerbated the situation.
- The yellow hat is the optimistic thinking mode, a logical approach to the things that went right and how the situation was handled well.
  - Often people find it more natural to wear either the black hat or the yellow hat so they may find it hard to work in the opposite thinking mode. This mode looks at the positives, the things that went right and made the situation better.
- The green hat is the creative thinking mode, and this is the opportunity to problem solve.
  - When reflecting on a learning experience, learners will need to identify what they could or should have done differently and therefore identify future learning needs and how they can be met. In doing this they could think creatively about possible action plans by taking into account how other people might have handled the situation.
- The blue hat is the organisational or reflective hat.
  - The order of the thinking hats is important and may change depending on the circumstances. So this should perhaps be the first hat to be worn. The learner

can order the hats according to the experience they have had. If they are very wound up or emotional about the situation they may need to vent first using the red hat. If they are very negative about an event perhaps the yellow hat could be used more than once. Use the blue hat to note down the order of hats that they think will work best. It can also be used at the end to evaluate the use of the hats and whether or not this order worked for this type of situation.

Thinking hats

Teach learners how to use de Bono's thinking hats as a mechanism to reflect on experiences that might result in challenging and conflicting thought processes. The parallel modes of thought will help learners to structure their thoughts and explore all aspects of the learning they will draw from their experience.

Skills, Reflective Observation (RO) 9: LM14

Being a follower

It is important to emphasise that leadership is not manipulation, it is not a covert attempt to make people do things they don't want to for the good of the company. Leadership is inclusive; it is about making people feel part of something positive, feel like they want to work to achieve the company goals. This may be because they actually agree with the objective or at the very least they are invested enough in their leader that they want to help them on their way to the goal. Leadership is not the boss on a secret mission to coerce the minions; we are part of the leadership process as leaders and as followers. As such we should be aware of ourselves as followers, be aware of the impact that the leadership process may have on us (*see* Figure 7.7). Other leaders, whether they are leaders by title or simply colleagues with natural leadership skills, will impact upon our perceptions – of the learning context, the nature of the knowledge and skills we are teaching, our opinions of our learners and indeed on our attitude to self-directedness.

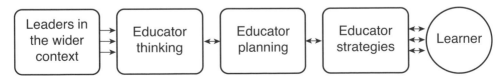

FIGURE 7.7 The impact of leadership on an educator's teaching (adapted from Ramsden)

> ### The impact of leadership
>
> Consider who the leaders are in your periphery and how their leadership might be impacting on your teaching and on your attitude to self-directedness. Be self-aware about the impact of external sources on your beliefs and actions and avoid the risk of your words, beliefs and actions being out of alignment. This would undermine your relationship with your learner.
>
> *Self-belief, Verbal Persuasion (VP) 8: LM15*

SUMMARY

This chapter on leadership and management has zoomed in from a wider organisational viewpoint to an individual level, taking in leadership and management tools that could be of use to us in building our pillars of skills, motivation and self-belief. It is perhaps fitting that the end of our hunt for bricks should be with a discussion of leadership as we deliberate on our vision for self-directedness in our context and consider how we can inspire our colleagues and learners towards it.

Before we finally wrap up we will revisit the overall model and draw together the bricks into the overarching structure so that we can see the full picture for the development of self-directed learners. While recapping the overall structure keep in mind the ideas of leadership that have been discussed here. We defined self-directedness in Chapter 2 and you will need to decide for yourself if this is congruent with your vision of self-directedness. You can flesh out this definition by considering the learning outcomes for each pillar and developing an overriding message for change. To make it happen you will not only need to develop leadership in your learner but also in yourself to ensure that self-directedness becomes embedded as a priority aim for your learner.

CHAPTER 8

Summary

If you have read every word so far, cover to (almost) cover, congratulations, that is no mean feat. If you have read the first chapter and skipped to the last then, without meaning to sound like your maths teacher telling you not to look up the homework answers in the back of the book, I strongly suggest that you use more than the brick titles. Use the codes embedded into each brick to turn back and add breadth and depth to your understanding of the brick before going any further.

THE THREE PILLAR MODEL OF SELF-DIRECTEDNESS

Before we progress into a summary of the bricks, let's just recap the model (*see* Figure 8.1).

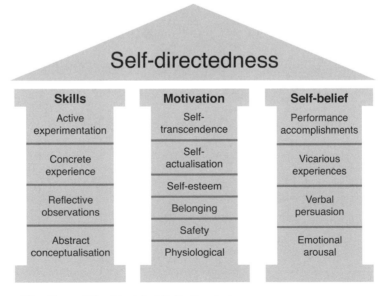

FIGURE 8.1 The Three Pillar Model of Self-directedness

There are three layers to the model, which allows it to be considered at a number of different levels. First is the overall structure in which self-directedness is held up by three pillars of skills, motivation and self-belief. To successfully develop self-directedness in learners we need to make sure each of these pillars is in place. Learners need to have:

- the learning skills necessary to successfully embark upon and complete learning activities and an understanding of their strengths and weaknesses in the learning process
- the motivation to take up learning opportunities and the insight into their personal motivators that will allow them to motivate themselves in the future
- the self-belief to pursue learning to completion despite obstacles and failures and the self-awareness to recognise events that might damage their level of self-belief.

These three factors provide the support necessary to develop self-directedness in our learners:

Self-directedness describes a learner who is able and willing to seek out learning opportunities and who holds the necessary belief in their own abilities to take control of their learning in formal and informal settings. They will identify suitable learning objectives given internal and external factors and work towards them in an effective manner using appropriate resources and strategies. They will then analyse, evaluate and reflect upon the outcomes of their learning in order to inform future learning opportunities.

The second layer of our model of self-directedness is the theory used to add depth and structure to each of our pillars. The Skills Pillar is structured around Kolb's Experiential Learning Cycle:

- concrete experience (CE)
- reflective observation (RO)
- abstract conceptualisation (AC)
- active experimentation (AE).

The Motivation Pillar uses Maslow's hierarchy of needs:

- physiological needs (P)
- safety needs (S)
- belongingness needs (B)
- self-esteem needs (SE)
- self-actualisation needs (SA)
- self-transcendence needs (ST).

The Self-belief Pillar is built around Bandura's theory of self-efficacy:

- performance accomplishments (PA)

- vicarious experience (VE)
- verbal persuasion (VP)
- emotional arousal (EA).

Finally, the third layer of the model is the one that will be different for each individual learner and context. This provides the bricks that are used to build up each of the categories within each pillar. The bricks that are relevant will need to be selected by the educator and used as appropriate to develop self-directedness. These bricks have been found throughout many different areas of literature and each is assigned a code (*see* Figure 8.2) to help us place it within the model and to find more information in this book. The first part of these codes tells us which pillar the brick belongs in (skills, motivation or self-belief), then the category (e.g. verbal persuasion is VP) and then the number of the brick within that category (e.g. VP3 is the third verbal persuasion brick).

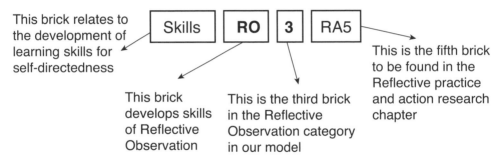

FIGURE 8.2 Coding the bricks

The second part of the code tells us which chapter the brick has been taken from and then the number of the brick within that chapter. So each chapter has been assigned a code:

- Self-directedness and Adult learning (SD)
- People and Places (PP)
- Mentoring and Coaching (MC)
- Learning and Teaching (LT)
- Reflective Practice and Action Research (RA)
- Leadership and Management (LM).

The next three tables summarise the bricks we have found for each of the pillars: the Skills Pillar, Table 8.1; the Motivation Pillar, Table 8.2; and the Self-belief Pillar, Table 8.3. For each pillar consider what the priorities are for your context and your learner. Use the codes to refer to the book and the original discussion of the related literature.

SKILLS PILLAR BRICKS

TABLE 8.1 A summary of the bricks in the Skills Pillar

Category	Brick title	Brick code
Concrete Experience	Maturity and professional readiness	Skills, CE1: SD1
Concrete Experience	Self-directed teaching	Skills, CE2: SD4
Concrete Experience	Transformational teaching	Skills, CE3: SD5
Concrete Experience	Learning styles	Skills, CE4: PP7
Concrete Experience	The learning environment	Skills, CE5: PP11
Concrete Experience	Reality of experience	Skills, CE6: RA5
Concrete Experience	Competences	Skills, CE7: LT3
Concrete Experience	The hidden curriculum	Skills, CE8: LT4
Concrete Experience	Objectives and outcomes	Skills, CE9: LT10
Concrete Experience	Diagnosing difficulties	Skills, CE10: LT22
Reflective Observation	Personality types	Skills, RO1: PP2
Reflective Observation	Emotional intelligence	Skills, RO2: PP3
Reflective observation	Perspectives on life	Skills, RO3: MC12
Reflective Observation	Negative automatic thoughts	Skills, RO4: MC17
Reflective observation	Deep reflective processes	Skills, RO5: RA4
Reflective Observation	The reflective conversation	Skills, RO6: RA6
Reflective Observation	High-level questioning	Skills, RO7: LT11
Reflective Observation	Critical self-assessment	Skills, RO8: LT12
Reflective Observation	Thinking hats	Skills, RO9: LM14
Abstract Conceptualisation	Creativity	Skills, AC1: PP5
Abstract Conceptualisation	A critical visioning approach	Skills, AC2: MC5
Abstract Conceptualisation	Open questioning	Skills, AC3: MC14
Abstract Conceptualisation	The learner as action researcher	Skills, AC4: RA12
Abstract Conceptualisation	Likelihood vs impact grid	Skills, AC5: LM5
Abstract Conceptualisation	Analysis and gut instinct	Skills, AC6: LM9
Active Experimentation	Virtual resources	Skills, AE1: PP15
Active Experimentation	Coaching conversation cones	Skills, AE2: MC10
Active Experimentation	Structuring the problem	Skills, AE3: MC11
Active Experimentation	A solution-focused approach	Skills, AE4: MC15
Active Experimentation	Habit loops	Skills, AE5: MC20
Active Experimentation	Assessment for Learning	Skills, AE6: LT5
Active Experimentation	Learners as leaders	Skills, AE7: LM6

MOTIVATION PILLAR BRICKS

TABLE 8.2 A summary of the bricks in the Motivation Pillar

Category	Brick title	Brick code
Self-Transcendence	Personal readiness	Motivation, ST1: SD2
Self-Transcendence	Critical reflection	Motivation, ST2: RA3
Self-Transcendence	Feedback on processing	Motivation, ST3: LT15
Self-Transcendence	Feedforward	Motivation, ST4: LT19
Self-Transcendence	Just surviving or at your best?	Motivation, ST5: LM8
Self-Transcendence	Operational capacity	Motivation, ST6: LM10
Self-Actualisation	The curriculum vs self-directedness	Motivation, SA1: SD6
Self-Actualisation	Type of learner	Motivation, SA2: PP8
Self-Actualisation	Positive learning atmosphere	Motivation, SA3: PP17
Self-Actualisation	Scaffolding	Motivation, SA4: LT2
Self-Actualisation	Problem-based learning	Motivation, SA5: LT8
Self-Actualisation	Teaching style	Motivation, SA6: LT9
Self-Actualisation	Feedback for high-flying learners	Motivation, SA7: LT25
Self-Actualisation	Organisational culture	Motivation, SA8: LM1
Self-Esteem	Physical locus of authority	Motivation, SE1: PP13
Self-Esteem	Faith in the learner's ability	Motivation, SE2: MC7
Self-Esteem	Active listening	Motivation, SE3: MC13
Self-Esteem	Supportive vs challenging feedback	Motivation, SE4: LT14
Self-Esteem	Seeking feedback	Motivation, SE5: LT21
Self-Esteem	Defensive responses to feedback	Motivation, SE6: LT24
Self-Esteem	Intrinsic or extrinsic motivation	Motivation, SE7: LM12
Belongingness	Empathy and understanding	Motivation, B1: PP4
Belongingness	Relationships	Motivation, B2: PP19
Belongingness	Developing rapport	Motivation, B3: MC8
Belongingness	Collaborative learning	Motivation, B4: LT7
Belongingness	The learning contract	Motivation, B5: LT23
Belongingness	Learning organisation	Motivation, B6: LM2
Safety	Stereotype threat	Motivation, S1: SD3
Safety	Feedback environment	Motivation, S2: PP14
Safety	The mentor–mentee relationship	Motivation, S3: MC3
Safety	Survival anxiety vs learning anxiety	Motivation, S4: LM4
Physiological	Learner environmental control	Motivation, P1: PP12
Physiological	Virtual access	Motivation, P2: PP16

SELF-BELIEF PILLAR BRICKS

TABLE 8.3 A summary of the bricks in the Self-belief Pillar

Category	Brick title	Brick code
Performance Accomplishments	Information overload	Self-belief, PA1: SD7
Performance Accomplishments	Congruent objectives	Self-belief, PA2: MC1
Performance Accomplishments	SMART targets	Self-belief, PA3: MC9
Performance Accomplishments	Transactional analysis	Self-belief, PA4: MC18
Performance Accomplishments	Positive reflection	Self-belief, PA5: RA2
Performance Accomplishments	The 3 H's	Self-belief, PA6: RA7
Performance Accomplishments	The objectives tree	Self-belief, PA7: RA9
Performance Accomplishments	Spacing and interleaving in curriculum planning	Self-belief, PA8: LT1
Performance Accomplishments	Learner specific feedback	Self-belief, PA9: LT17
Performance Accomplishments	Amount of feedback	Self-belief, PA10: LT18
Performance Accomplishments	Delivering the outcome	Self-belief, PA11: LM7
Vicarious Experience	Learning for all	Self-belief, VE1: PP18
Vicarious Experience	The modelling mentor	Self-belief, VE2: MC4
Vicarious Experience	Modelling reflective practice	Self-belief, VE3: RA10
Vicarious Experience	The educator as action researcher	Self-belief, VE4: RA11
Vicarious Experience	Modelling leadership	Self-belief, VE5: LM13
Verbal Persuasion	Growable intelligence	Self-belief, VP1: PP9
Verbal Persuasion	Credibility	Self-belief, VP2: PP10
Verbal Persuasion	Awareness of mentoring	Self-belief, VP3: MC2
Verbal Persuasion	A confident educator	Self-belief, VP4: MC6
Verbal Persuasion	Formative feedback	Self-belief, VP5: LT13
Verbal Persuasion	Feedback on judgements	Self-belief, VP6: LT16
Verbal Persuasion	Power bases	Self-belief, VP7: LM11
Verbal Persuasion	The impact of leadership	Self-belief, VP8: LM15
Emotional Arousal	Berne's ego states	Self-belief, EA1: PP1
Emotional Arousal	Stress and hassles	Self-belief, EA2: PP6
Emotional Arousal	Individuality vs community	Self-belief, EA3: MC16
Emotional Arousal	Visualisation	Self-belief, EA4: MC19
Emotional Arousal	Emotional reflection	Self-belief, EA5: RA1
Emotional Arousal	The CIA framework	Self-belief, EA6: RA8
Emotional Arousal	A strategic approach	Self-belief, EA7: LT6
Emotional Arousal	Receiving feedback	Self-belief, EA8: LT20
Emotional Arousal	Change responses	Self-belief, EA9: LM3

USING THE MODEL

We have now brought together the bricks to help develop self-directedness in our learners. To attempt to work on all of these at once would be impossible, so use the structure of this model as a tool to audit your current practice and the specific needs of your current learner(s). Consider the outcomes identified for each pillar in Chapter 1: which ones do you feel you are achieving? Which ones do you feel need work? This will help you work out which pillar and which bricks you should focus your efforts on first as you develop a teaching style and a learning environment that cultivates self-directedness in your learners.

FINAL WORDS

We are all part of a healthcare context that has been undergoing constant change since inception and needs to evolve further to meet current demands let alone the unknown and unpredictable future challenges our learners will face.

> The greatest demand placed on the NHS comes from people with long term conditions rather than acute ones. They need continuing help to look after themselves, manage intermittent crises and maintain their health. Despite many excellent examples to the contrary, the NHS is still a service that is geared more towards one-off episodes of treatment. It needs to change so as to adapt to the new reality and, most profoundly of all, we need to begin to treat the NHS as what it is – a part of the local infrastructure and services that we all rely on. It should not be seen as a completely separate activity or industry but part of the network of organisations and services locally that help elderly, disabled and sick people to get on with their lives, children to develop, our streets to be safe and our environment and workplaces clean and healthy.[1]

In a workplace where standing still is moving backwards, change is the one constant in healthcare. Evidence-based medicine still feels relatively new (in the grand scheme of medicine) and yet there is now emerging a new culture of values-based medicine. The patient has been increasingly part of the process at the front line of medicine, but patient groups and patient representatives are becoming valuable members of the behind-the-scenes staff. They are involved in patient participation groups (PPGs), clinical commissioning groups (CCGs) and faculty boards, in planning care pathways and in education as a resource but also as teachers, organisers and examiners. The rapidly changing landscape of medicine and therefore of medical education makes the requirement for self-direction in learning even greater. Much of the content that your learners take away with them will be out of date in 10 years' time. You know this of course, sorry to remind you of such a depressing truth. But worry not, the skills you help them acquire, the insight into their learning and motivations you help them develop and the belief they have in their ability to cope in this environment will be the legacy you leave them with. That is definitely worth it.

References

CHAPTER 1: A MODEL FOR SELF-DIRECTEDNESS

1. Team Sky. Aggregation of Marginal Gains. BSkyB; 2014. Available at: www.teamsky.com/article/0,27290,17547_5792058,00.html#B0cr1PsHByhDZ12f.97 (accessed 21 August 2014).
2. Dewey J. *Democracy and Education*. New York, NY: The Free Press: Simon & Schuster Inc.; 1944.
3. Health Education England. *The Delivery of 21st Century Services: the implications for the evolution of the healthcare science workforce*. London: National Health Service; 2014.
4. Knowles M. *The Adult Learner: a neglected species*. Houston, Tx: Gulf Publishing Company; 1973.
5. Kolb DA. *Experiential Learning: experience as the source of learning and development*. Englewood Cliffs, NJ: Prentice Hall; 1984.
6. Brookfield SD. *Adult Learners, Adult Education and the Community*. Milton Keynes: Open University Press; 1983.
7. Kelly G. *The Psychology of Personal Constructs*. New York, NY: Norton; 1955.
8. Bringuier JC, Piaget J. *Conversations with Jean Piaget*. Chicago, IL: University of Chicago Press; 1980.
9. Maslow AH. A theory of human motivation. *Psychological Review*. 1943 July; **50**(4): 370–96.
10. Maslow AH. *The Farther Reaches of Human Nature*. London: Penguin Books Ltd; 1976.
11. Koltko-Rivera ME. Rediscovering the later version of Maslow's Hierachy of Needs: self-transcendence and opportunities for theory, research and unification. *Review of General Psychology*. 2006; **10**(4): 302–17.
12. Hofstede G. The cultural relativity of the quality of life concept. *The Academy of Management Review*. 1984 July; **9**(3): 389–98.
13. Wahba MA, Bridwell LG. Maslow reconsidered: a review of research on the Need Hierachy Theory. *Organisational Behaviour and Human Performance*. 1976; **15**(2): 212–40.
14. Vroom VH. *Work and Motivation*. San Francisco, CA: Jossey-Bass Inc.; 1995.
15. Bandura A. Self-efficacy: toward a unifying theory of behavioral change. *Psychological Review*. 1977; **84**(2): 191–215.
16. Sabbaghian ZS. *Adult Self-Directedness and Self-Concept: an exploration of relationship* [dissertation]. Ames, IA: Iowa State University; 1980.
17. Singh PB. *The Relationship Between Group Empowerment and Self-Directed Learning in Selected Small Groups in Michigan*. East Lansing, MI: Michigan State University; 1993.

CHAPTER 2: SELF-DIRECTEDNESS AND ADULT LEARNING

1. Grow GO. Teaching learners to be self-directed. *Adult Education Quarterly*. 1991; **41**(3): 125–49.
2. Merriam S, Caffarella RS. *Learning in Adulthood*. 2nd ed. San Francisco, CA: Jossey-Bass; 1999.
3. Candy PC. *Self-direction for Lifelong Learning: a comprehensice guide to theory and practice*. San Francisco, CA: Jossey-Bass; 1991.
4. Garrison DR. Self-directed learning: toward a comprehensive model. *Adult Education Quarterly*. 1997; **48**(1): 18–33.
5. Brockett R, Hiemstra R. *Self-Direction in Adult Learning: perspectives on theory, research and practice*. London: Routledge; 1991.
6. Knowles M. *The Adult Learner: a neglected species*. Houston: Gulf Publishing Company; 1973.
7. Knowles M. *Self-directed Learning: a guide for learners and teachers*. London: Prentice-Hall International (UK Ltd.); 1975.
8. Brookfield SD. *Adult Learning: an overview*. In: Tuinjman A, editor. *International Encyclopaedia of Education*. Oxford: Pergamon Press; 1995. Available at: www.ict.mic.ul.ie/adult_ed/overview.htm (accessed 8 August 2014).
9. Hammond M, Collins R. *Self-Directed Learning: critical practice*. London: Kogan Page; 1991.
10. Cox K. Persuading colleagues to change: fifteen lessons learned from more than 20 years trying. *Education for Health*. 1999 November; **12**(3): 347–54.
11. Vygotsky LS. *Mind in Society: the development of higher psychological processes*. Cole M, John-Steiner V, Scribner S, Souberman E, editors. London: Harvard University Press; 1978.
12. Demetriou A, Spanoudis G, Mouyi A. Educating the developing mind: towards an overarching paradigm. *Educational Psychology Review*. 2011; **23**: 601–63.
13. Long HB, Agyekum SK. Guglielmino's self-directed learning readiness scale: a validation study. *Higher Education*. 1983; **12**: 77–87.
14. McCarthy WF. *The Self-Directedness and Attitude Toward Mathematics of Younger and Older Undergraduate Mathematics Students* [dissertation]. Syracuse, NY: Syracuse University; 1985.
15. Guglielmino LM. *Development of the Self-Directed Learning Readiness Scale* [dissertation]. Athens, GA: University of Georgia; 1977.
16. Mourad SA. *The Relationship of Grade Level, Sex, and Creativity to Readiness for Self-Directed Learning Among Intellectually Gifted Students* [dissertation]. Athens, GA: University of Georgia; 1979.
17. Sabbaghian ZS. *Adult Self-Directedness and Self-Concept: an exploration of relationship* [dissertation]. Ames, IA: Iowa State University; 1980.
18. Hassan AJ. *An Investigation of the Learning Projects of Adults of High and Low Readiness for Self-Direction Learning* [dissertation]. Iowa, IA: Iowa State University; 1981.
19. Lacey CL. *Readiness for Self-Directed Learning in Women During Four Stages of Pregnancy* [dissertation]. Columbia, MO: University of Missouri; 1988.
20. Field L. An investigation into the structure, validity, and reliability of Guglielmino's Self-Directed Learning Readiness Scale. *Adult Education Quarterly*. 1989; **39**: 125–39.
21. Deakin Crick R, Broadfoot P, Claxton G. Developing an Effective Lifelong Learning Inventory: the ELLI Project. *Assessment in Education*. 2004; **11**(3): 247–73.
22. Furlong J, Maynard T. *Mentoring Student Teachers*. London: Rutledge; 1995.

23. Gavriel G, Gavriel J. Professional growth of trainees: applying teacher training models to the teaching of GPs. *British Journal of General Practice.* 2011; **61**(591): 630–2.

24. Newman P, Peile E. Valuing learners' experience and supporting further growth: educational models to help experienced adult learners in medicine. *British Medical Journal.* 2002 July; **325**: 200–2.

25. Mahoney M. Adverse baggage in the learning environment. In: Hiemstra R, editor. *Creating Environments for Effective Adult Learning.* San Francisco, CA: Jossey-Bass; 1991. pp. 51–60.

26. Kübler-Ross E. *On Death and Dying.* New York, NY: Scribner; 1969.

27. Rogers A, Horrocks N. *Teaching Adults.* 4th ed. Maidenhead: McGraw Hill & Open University Press; 2010.

28. Kai J, Beavan J, Faull C, *et al.* Professional uncertainty and disempowerment responding to ethnic diversity in health care: a qualitative study. *PLoS Med.* 2007; **4**(11): 1766–75.

29. Appel M, Kronberger N. Stereotypes and the achievement gap: stereotype threat prior to test taking. *Educational Psychology Review.* 2012; **24**: 609–35.

30. Schmader T, Johns M, Forbes C. An integrated process model of stereotype threat effects on performance. *Psychological Review.* 2008; **115**: 336–56.

31. Thoman DB, Smith JL, Brown ER, *et al.* Beyond performance: a motivational experiences model of stereotype threat. *Educational Psychology Review.* 2013 June; **25**(2): 211–43.

32. Gibbons M. *The Self-Directed Learning Handbook.* San Francisco: Jossey-Bass; 2002.

33. Slavich GM, Zimbardo PG. Transformational teaching: theoretical underpinnings, basic principles, and core methods. *Educational Psychology Review.* 2012; **24**: 569–608.

34. Piskurich GM. *Self-Directed Learning: a practical guide to design, develpement, and implementation.* San Francisco: Jossey-Bass Inc.; 1993.

35. Brookfield SD. *Understanding and Facilitating Adult Learning.* Milton Keynes: Open University Press; 1986.

36. Andersen LW. What every teacher should know: reflecting on 'Educating the Developing Mind'. *Educational Psychology Review.* 2012; **24**: 13–18.

CHAPTER 3: PEOPLE AND PLACES

1. Lewin K. *A Dynamic Theory of Personality: selected papers.* London: McGraw-Hill Book Company, Inc.; 1935.

2. Kluckhohn C, Murray HA. Personality formation: the determinants. In: Kluckhohn C, Murray HA, Schneider DM, editors. *Personality in Nature, Society and Culture.* 2nd ed. New York, NY: Alfred A. Knopf; 1953. pp. 53–70.

3. Freud S. *The Standard Edition of the Complete Psychological Works of Sigmund Freud: Volume XIX (1923–1925).* Strachey J, editor. London: Vintage; 2001.

4. Berne E. *Games People Play: the psychology of human relationships.* London: Penguin Books; 1968.

5. Northouse PG. *Leadership: theory and practice.* 5th ed. London: Sage Publications Ltd; 2010.

6. Eysenck HJ. *Dimensions of Personality.* New Brunswick, NJ: Transaction Publishers; 1998.

7. Myers and Briggs Foundation. The Myers & Briggs Foundation. Available at: www.myers briggs.org/my-mbti-personality-type/mbti-basics/ (accessed 21 August 2014).

8. Goleman D. *Working with Emotional Intelligence.* New York, NY: Bantamdell; 1998.

9. Mayer JD, Salovey P, Caruso DR, Sitarenios G. Measuring emotional intelligence with the MSCEIT V2.0. *Emotion.* 2003; **3**(1): 97–105.

10. Toubia O. Idea generation, creativity, and incentives. *Marketing Science*. 2006 September/ Octber; **25**(5): 411–25.

11. Shackleton V, Fletcher C. *Individual Differences: theories and applications*. London: Methuen & Co. Ltd.; 1984.

12. Biggs J, Tang C. *Teaching for Quality Learning at University*. 3rd ed. Maidenhead: Open University Press; 2007.

13. Holmes TH, Rahe RH. The social readjustment ratings scale. *Journal of Psychosomatic Research*. 1967 August; **11**(2): 213–18.

14. Kanner AD, Cyne JC, Schaefer C, *et al.* Comparison of two modes of stress measurement: daily hassles and uplifts versus major life events. *Journal of Behavioral Medicine*. 1981 March; **4**(1): 1–39.

15. Goulding J, Syed-Khuzzan S. A study on the validity of a four-variant diagnostic learning styles questionnaire. *Education & Training*. 2014; **56**(2/3): 141–64.

16. Fleming ND, Mills C. Not another inventory, rather a catalyst for reflection. *To Improve the Academy*. 1992 January; **11**: 137–55.

17. Honey P, Mumford A. *The Learning Style's Helper Guide*. Maidenhead: Peter Honey Publications; 2006.

18. Kolb DA. *Experiential Learning: experience as the source of learning and development*. Englewood Cliffs, NJ: Prentice Hall; 1984.

19. Houle CO. The inquiring mind. *Adult Education Quarterly*. 1961; **13**: 122–3.

20. Glock S, Kovacs C. Educational psychology: using insights from implicit attitude measures. *Educational Psychology Review*. 2013 December; **25**(4): 503–22.

21. Mangels JA, Butterfield B, Lamb J, *et al.* Why do beliefs about intelligence influence learning success? A social cognitive neuroscience model. *Social Cognitive and Affective Neuroscience*. 2006; **1**: 75–86.

22. Herrnstein RJ, Murray C. *The Bell Curve: intelligence and class structure in American life*. New York, NY: The Free Press; 1994.

23. Brookfield SD. *The Skillful Teacher*. San Francisco, CA: Jossey-Bass; 2000.

24. Hiemstra R. Aspects of effective learning environments. In: Hiemstra R, editor. *Creating Environments for Effective Adult Learning*. San Francisco, CA: Jossey-Bass; 1991. pp. 5–12.

25. Fulton RD. A conceptual model for understanding the physical attributes of learning environments. In: Hiemstra R, editor. *Creating Environments for Effective Ault Learning*. San Francisco, CA: Jossey-Bass; 1991. pp. 13–22.

26. Starr J. *The Coaching Manual: the definitive guide to the process, principles and skills of personal coaching*. 3rd ed. Harlow: Pearson Education Limited; 2011.

27. OFSTED. *Virtual Learning Environments: an evaluation of their development in a sample of educational settings*. London: The Office for Standards in Education, Children's Services and Skills (OFSTED); 2009. Report No.: 070251.

28. Winters FI, Greens JA, Costich CM. Self-regulation of learning within computer-based learning environments: a critical analysis. *Educational Psychology Review*. 2008 July; **20**: 429–44.

29. Kelly GA. *The Psychology of Personal Constructs Volume 2: Clinical diagnosis and psychotherapy*. London: Routledge; 1991.

30. Bandura A. Self-efficacy: toward a unifying theory of behavioral change. *Psychological Review*. 1977; **84**(2): 191–215.

31. Hiemstra R, Sisco B. *Individualizing Instruction: making learning personal, empowering, and successful.* San Francisco, CA: Jossey-Bass; 1991.

CHAPTER 4: MENTORING AND COACHING

1. Wheatley MJ. Partnering with confusion and uncertainty. Shambhala Sun. 2001 November. Available at: www.margaretwheatley.com/articles/partneringwithconfusion.html (accessed 21 August 2014).
2. Parsloe E, Leedham M. *Coaching and Mentoring: practical conversations to improve learning.* 2nd ed. London: Kogan-Page; 2009.
3. Gallwey WT. *The Inner Game of Work.* New York, NY: Random House Trade Paperbacks; 2000.
4. Greene J, Grant AM. *Solution Focused Coaching.* Harlow: Pearson Education Limited; 2003.
5. Bayley H, Chambers R, Donovan C. *The Good Mentoring Toolkit for Healthcare.* Oxford: Radcliffe Publishing; 2004.
6. Tulpa C. Coaching within organisations. In: Passmore J, editor. *Excellence in Coaching: the industry guide.* London: Kogan-Page; 2006. pp. 26–43.
7. Anderson EM, Shannon AL. Toward a conceptualisation of mentoring. In: Kerry T, Mayes AS, editors. *Issues in Mentoring.* London: Routledge; 1995. pp. 25–34.
8. Watkins C. Developing effective mentoring. In: McIntyre D, Hagger H, editors. *Mentoring in Initial Teacher Education.* London: Paul Hamlyn Foundation; 1994.
9. Golian LM, Galbraith MW. Effective mentoring programs for professional library development. In: Williams D, Garten E, editors. *Advances in Library Administration and Organisation Volume 14.* Greenwich CT: Jai Press; 1994. pp. 95–124. Cited in: Galbraith MW. Mentoring toward self-directedness. *Adult Learning.* 2003 September; **14**: pp. 9–11.
10. Shea GF. *Mentoring: how to develop successful mentor behaviours.* Menlo Park, CA: Crisp Publications; 2002.
11. Cohen NH. *Mentoring Adult Learners: a guide for educators and trainers (professional practices).* Malabar, FL: Krieger Publishing Company; 1995.
12. Alexander G, Renshaw B. *Supercoaching: the missing ingredient for high performance.* London: Random House Business Books; 2005.
13. Laborde G. *Influencing with Integrity: management skills for communication and negotiation.* Carmarthen: Crown House Publishing Ltd.; 1983.
14. Locke EA, Latham GP. Building a practically useful theory of goal setting and task motivation: a thirty-five year odyssey. *The American Psychologist.* 2002 September; **56**(9): 705–17.
15. Alexander G. Behavioural coaching: the GROW Model. In: Passmore J, editor. *Excellence in Coaching: the industry guide.* London: Kogan Page Limited; 2006. pp. 61–72.
16. Nichols R. Factors in listening comprehension. *Speech Monographs.* 1948; **15**(2): 154–63.
17. Bresser F, Wilson C. What is coaching? In: Passmore J, editor. *Excellence in Coaching: the industry guide.* London: Kogan Page Limited; 2006. pp. 9–25.
18. Brownell J. *Listening: Attitude, Principles, and Skills.* 3rd ed. Boston, MA: Allyn & Bacon; 2005.
19. Whitmore J. *Coaching for Performance.* 4th ed. London: Nicholas Brealey; 2009.
20. Costa A. John Hopkins University. [Online]; 2001. Available at: education.jhu.edu/PD/newhorizons/strategies/topics/Cognitive%20Coaching/ (accessed 22 August 2014).

21. Ellison J, Hayes C. Cognitive coaching. In: Knight J, editor. *Coaching: approaches and perspectives*. Thousand Oak, CA: Corwin Press; 2009. pp. 70–90.

22. Berne E. *Games People Play: the psychology of human relationships*. London: Penguin Books; 1968.

23. Martin N. *Habit: the 95% of behaviour marketers ignore*. Upper Saddle River, NJ: Pearson Education, Inc.; 2008.

24. Graybiel AM. Habits, rituals, and evaluative brain. *Annual Review of Neuroscience*. 2008; **31**: 359–87.

CHAPTER 5: REFLECTIVE PRACTICE AND ACTION RESEARCH

1. Dewey J. *Democracy and Education*. New York: The Free Press: Simon & Schuster Inc.; 1944.

2. Schön DA. *Educating the Reflective Practitioner*. San Francisco: Jossey-Bass Inc.; 1987.

3. Dinsmore DL, Alexander PA, Loughlin SM. Focusing the conceptual lens on metacognition, self-regulation, and self-regulated learning. *Educational Psychology Review*. 2008; **20**: 391–409.

4. Fox E, Riconscente M. Metacognition and self-regulation in James, Piaget, and Vygotsky. *Educational Psychology Review*. 2008; **20**: 373–89.

5. Ashcroft K, Foerman-Peck L. *Managing Teaching and Learning in Further and Higher Education*. London: RoutledgeFalmer; 1994.

6. Boud D, Keogh R, Walker D. Promoting reflection in learning: a model. In: Boud D, Keogh R, Walker D, editors. *Reflection: turning experience into learning*. Abingdon: Routledge; 1985. pp. 18–40.

7. Shulman LS. Knowledge and teaching: foundations of the new reform. *Harvard Educational Review*. 1987 February; **57**(1): 1–22.

8. Moon JA. *Reflection in Learning and Professional Development: theory and practice*. Abingdon: RoutledgeFalmer; 1999.

9. Atkins S, Kathy M. Reflection: a review of the literature. *Journal of Advanced Nursing*. 1993; **18**: 1188–92.

10. Graybiel AM. Habits, rituals, and evaluative brain. *Annual Review of Neuroscience*. 2008; **31**: 359–87.

11. Brookfield SD. *Adult Learning: an overview*. In: Tuinjman A, editor. *International Encyclopaedia of Education*. Oxford: Pergamon Press; 1995. Available at: www.ict.mic.ul.ie/adult_ed/overview.htm (accessed 8 August 2014).

12. King PM, Kitchener KS. *Developing Reflective Judgement*. San Francisco, CA: Jossey-Bass; 1994.

13. Mezirow J. A critical theory of adult learning and education. *Adult Education*. 1981 Fall; **32**(1): 3–24.

14. Loughran JJ. Effective reflective practice: in search of meaning in learning about teaching. *Journal of Teacher Education*. 2002; **53**(1): 33–43.

15. Johns C. *Becoming a Reflectice Practitioner*. 4th ed. Chichester: John Wiley & Sons, Ltd.; 2013.

16. Dinsmore DL, Alexander PA. A critical discussion of deep and surface processing: what it means, how it is measured, the role of context, and model specification. *Educational Psychology Review*. 2012; **24**: 499–567.

17. Argyris C, Schön DA. *Theory in Practice: increasing professional effectiveness.* San Francisco: Jossey-Bass Inc.; 1974.

18. Bringuier JC, Piaget J. *Conversations with Jean Piaget.* Chicago: University of Chicago Press; 1980.

19. Habermas J. *Knowledge and Human Interests.* Boston, MA: Beacon Press; 1971. Cited in: Mezirow J. A critical theory of adult learning and education. *Adult Education.* 1981 Fall; **32**(1): 3–24.

20. McNiff J, Lomax P, Whitehead J. *You and Your Action Research Project.* 2nd ed. Abingdon: RoutledgeFalmer; 2003.

21. Gibbs G. *Learning by Doing: a guide to teaching and learning methods.* Oxford: Further Education Unit. Oxford Polytechnic; 1988.

22. Borton T. Reach, *Touch, and Teach: student concerns and process education.* New York, NY: McGraw-Hill Paperbacks; 1970.

23. Driscoll J. *Practising Clinical Supervision: a reflective approach for healthcare professionals.* 2nd ed. Edinburgh: Bailliere Tindall; 2007.

24. Honey P, Mumford A. *The Learning Style's Helper Guide.* Maidenhead: Peter Honey Publications; 2006.

25. Thompson S, Thompson N. *The Critically Reflective Practitioner.* New York: Palgrave MacMillan; 2008.

26. Van Manen M. Linking ways of knowing with ways of being practical. *Curriculum Inquiry.* 1977; **6**(3): 205–28.

27. Hart E, Bond M. *Action Research for Health and Social Care: a guide to practice.* Buckingham: Open University Press; 1995.

28. Whitehead J. *The Growth of Educational Knowledge: creating your own living educational theories.* Bournemouth: Hyde; 1993.

29. Kemmis S, McTaggart R. Participatory Action Research: communicative action and the public shere. In: Denzin NK, Lincoln Y, editors. *Strategies of Qualitative Inquiry.* 3rd ed. London: Sage Publications Inc.; 2008. pp. 271–330.

30. Kolb DA. *Experiential Learning: experience as the source of learning and development.* Englewood Cliffs, NJ: Prentice Hall; 1984.

31. Zeichner KM. Action Research: personal renewal and social reconstruction. *Educational Action Research.* 1993; **1**(2): 199–219.

CHAPTER 6: LEARNING AND TEACHING

1. Knowles M. *The Adult Learner: a neglected species.* Houston, TX: Gulf Publishing Company; 1973.

2. Karpicke JD, Grimaldi PJ. Retrieval-based learning: a perspective for enhancing meaningful learning. *Educational Psychology Review.* 2012; **24**: 401–18.

3. Neary M. *Teaching, Assessing and Evaluation for Clinical Competence: a practical guide for practitioners and teachers.* Cheltenham: Nelson Thornes Ltd.; 2000.

4. Bruner J. *The Process of Education: a landmark in educational theory.* London: Harvard University Press; 1960.

5. Carpenter SK, Cepeda NJ, Rohrer D, *et al.* Using spacing to enhance diverse forms of learning: review of recent research and implications for instruction. *Educational Psychology Review.* 2012; **24**: 369–78.

6. Son LK, Simon DA. Distributive learning: data, metacognition, and educational implications. *Educational Psychology Review*. 2012; **24**: 379–99.

7. Rohrer D. Interleaving helps students distinguish amongst similar concepts. *Educational Psychology Review*. 2012; **24**: 355–67.

8. Biggs JB, Collis KF. *Evaluating the Quality of Learning: the SOLO taxonomy*. New York: Academic Press; 1982. Cited in: Biggs J, Tang C. *Teaching for Quality Learning at University*. 3rd ed. Maidenhead: Open University Press; 2007.

9. Vygotsky LS. *Mind in Society: the development of higher psychological processes*. Cole M, John-Steiner V, Scribner S, *et al.*, editors. London: Harvard University Press; 1978.

10. Belland BR. Distrbuted cognition as a lens to understand the effects of scaffolds: the role of transfer of responsibility. *Educational Psychology Review*. 2011; **23**: 577–600.

11. Hutchins E. *Cognition in the Wild*. Cambridge, MA: MIT Press; 1995.

12. Van der Pol J, Volman M, Veishuizen J. Scaffolding in teacher–student interaction: a decade of research. *Educational Psychlogy Review*. 2010; **22**: 271–96.

13. Jones E, Voorhees RA, Paulson K. *Defining and Assessing Learning: exploring competency-based initiatives*. Washington, D.C.: U.S. Department of Education, National Center for Education Statistics; 2001.

14. Voorhees RA. Competency-based learning models: a necessary future. *New Directions for Institutional Research*. 2001 **Summer**(110): 5–13.

15. Dreyfus H, Dreyfus S. *Mind Over Machine: the power of human intuition and expertise in the era of the computer*. New York, NY: The Free Press; 1986.

16. Harden RM. Planning a curriculum. In: Dent JA, Harden RM, editors. *A Practical Guide for Medical Teachers*. Churchill Livingstone; 2001. pp. 13–24.

17. Rawson KA, Dunlosky J. When is practice testing most effective for improving the durability and efficiency of student learning. *Educational Psychology Review*. 2012; **24**: 419–35.

18. Black P, Wiliam D. *Inside the Black Box*. London: GL Assessment Limited; 1998.

19. Department for Children, Schools and Families. *The Assessment for Learning Strategy*. London: Department for Children, Schools and Families; National Strategies; QCA; Chartered Institute of Educational Assessors; 2008. Report No.: 978-1-84775-147-8.

20. Gavriel J. Assessment for learning: a wider (classroom-researched) perspective is important for formative assessment and self-directed learning in general practice. *Education for Primary Care*. 2013; **24**: 93–6.

21. Looney JW. Integrating formative and summative assessment: progress toward a seamless system? *OECD Education Working Papers*. 2011; **58**. OECD Publishing.

22. Stiggins R. From formative assessment to Assessment FOR Learning: a path to success in standards-based schools. *Phi Delta Kappan*. 2005 December; **87**(4): 324–8.

23. Clark I. Formative assessment: assessment is for self-regulated learning. *Educational Psychology Review*. 2012; **24**: 205–49.

24. Barrows HS, Tamblyn RM. *Problem-Based Learning: an approach to medical education*. New York, NY: Springer Publishing Company, Inc.; 1998.

25. Poikela E, Nummenmaa AR. *Understanding Problem-Based Learning*. Tampere: Tampere University Press; 2006.

26. Adhicari M. A condensed problem-based learning format in clinical perinatology. *Education for Health*. 1998 November; **11**(3): 337–41.

27. O'Neill PA. Problem-Based Learning alongside clinical experience: reform of the Manchester curriculum. *Education for Health*. 1998 March; **11**(1): 37–48.

28. West SA. Objectives in response to students' uncertainty in a preclinical problem-based learning curriculum. *Education for Health.* 1998 November; **11**(3): 343–7.

29. Kaufman DM. Problem-Based Learning: time to step back? *Medical Education.* 2000; **34**: 510–11.

30. Rothman AI. Problem-Based Learning: time to move forward? *Medical Education.* 2000; **34**: 509–10.

31. Margetson D. What counts as Problem-Based Learning? *Education for Health.* 1998 July; **11**(2): 193–201.

32. Kelly D, Wykurz G. Patients as teachers: a new perspective in medical education. *Education for Health.* 1998 November; **11**(3): 369–77.

33. Maudsley G, Strivens J. Promoting professional knowledge, experiential learning and critical thinking for medical students. *Medical Education.* 2000; **34**: 535–44.

34. Loyens SMM, Magda J, Rikers RMJP. Self-directed learning in problem-based learning and its relationships with self-regulated learning. *Educational Psychology Review.* 2008; **20**: 411–27.

35. Hung W. The 3C3R Model: a conceptual framework for designing problems in PBL. *The Interdisciplinary Journal of Problem-based Learning.* 2006 Spring; **1**(1): 55–77.

36. Barrett T, Moore S, editors. *New Approaches to Problem-Based Learning: revitalising your practice in higher education.* Abingdon: Routledge; 2011.

37. Barrett T. *Students' Talk About Problem-Based Learning Liminal Spaces* [unpublished doctorate thesis]. Coventry: Coventry University; 2008. Cited in: Barrett T, Moore S, editors. *New Approaches to Problem-Based Learning: revitalising your practice in higher education.* Abingdon: Routledge; 2011.

38. Savin-Baden M, Howell Major C. *Foundations of Problem-Based-Learning.* Maidenhead: Open University Press; 2004.

39. Entwistle NJ, Ramsden P. *Understanding Student Learning.* New York, NY: Nichols Publihing Company; 1982.

40. Fleming ND, Mills C. Not another inventory, rather a catalyst for reflection. *To Improve the Academy.* 1992 January; **11**: 137–55.

41. Honey P, Mumford A. *The Learning Style's Helper Guide.* Maidenhead: Peter Honey Publications; 2006.

42. Grow GO. Teaching learners to be self-directed. *Adult Education Quarterly.* 1991; **41**(3): 125–49.

43. Wiliam D. *Embedded Formative Assessment.* Bloomington, IN: Solution Tree Press; 2011.

44. Gadsby C. *Perfect Assessment for Learning.* Beere J, editor. Carmarthen: Crown House Publishing Ltd; 2012.

45. Black P, Harrison C, Lee C, *et al. Assessment for Learning: putting it into practice.* Maidenhead: Open University Press; 2003.

46. Rowe MB. Wait time: slowing down may be a way of speeding up! *Journal of Teacher Education.* 1986 January/February; **37**: 43–50.

47. Smith I. *Asking Better Questions.* Cambridge: Cambridge Education; 2008.

48. Barnett JE, Francis AL. Using higher order thinking questions to foster critical thinking: a classroom study. *Educational Psychology.* 2012; **32**(2): 201.

49. Bloom BS *et al.* 1956. Cited in: Krathwohl DR, Bloom BS, Masia, BB *Taxonomy of Educational Objectives: the classification of educational goals. Handbook II: the affective domain.* New York: David McKay; 1964.

50. Krathwohl DR, Bloom BS, Masia, BB *Taxonomy of Educational Objectives: the classification of educational goals. Handbook II: the affective domain.* New York: David McKay; 1964.

51. Brown NJS, Wilson M. A model of cognition: the missing cornerstone of assessment. *Educational Psychology Review.* 2011; **23**: 221–34.

52. De Bono E. *De Bono's Thinking Course.* London: BBC Books; 1982.

53. Smith I. *Promoting Assessment by Pupils.* Cambridge: Cambridge Education; 2008.

54. Sadler DR. Formative assessment and the design of instructional systems. *Instructional Science.* 1989; **18**: 119–44.

55. Page EB. Teacher comments and student performance: a seventy-four classroom exeriment in school motivation. *Journal of Educational Psychology.* 1958 August; **49**(4): 173–81.

56. Butler R. Enhancing and undermining intrinsic motivation: the effects of task-involving and ego-involving evaluation on interest and performance. *British Journal of Educational Psychology.* 1988; **58**: 1–14.

57. Daloz LA. *Mentor: guiding the journey of adult learners.* 2nd ed. San Francisco, CA: Jossey-Bass; 2012.

58. Luft J. The Johari Window: a graphic model of awareness in interpersonal relations. *Human Relations Training News.* 1961; **5**(1): 6–7.

59. Purves AC. The teacher as reader: an anatomy. *College English.* 1984 March; **46**(3): 259–65.

60. Tang R. Do we allow what we encourage? How students are positioned by teacher feedback. *Australian Journal of Language and Literacy.* 2000 June; **23**(2): 157–68.

61. Glover C, Brown E. Written feedback for students: too much, too detailed or too incomprehensible to be effective? *Bioscience Education.* 2006; **7**(3).

62. Hattie J, Timperley H. The power of feedback. *Review of Educational Research.* 2007 March; **77**(1): 81–112.

63. Russell T. *Effective Feedback Skills.* 2nd ed. London: Kogan Page Limited; 1998.

64. Kulhavy RW, Stock WA. Feedback in writen instruction: the place of response certitude. *Educational Psychology Review.* 1989 December; **1**(4): 279–308.

65. Tan SH, Pang JS. Sticks and stones will break my bones but failure feedback may not hurt me: gender differences in the relationship between achievement motive, coping strategies and environmental mastery. *Educational Psychology Review.* 2012; **32**(3): 373–88.

66. Pfeiffer JW, Jones JE. Openness, collusion, and feedback. In: Pfeiffer JW, Jones JE, editors. *The 1979 Annual Handbook for Group Facilitators.* San Diego, CA: University Associates; 1972. Cited in: Jones JE, Bearley W. *360° Feedback: strategies, tactics, and techniques for developing leaders.* Amherst, MA: HRD Press; 1996.

67. Pendleton D, Schofield T, Tate P, *et al. The New Consultation: developing doctor–patient communication.* Oxford: Oxford University Press; 2003.

68. King J. Giving feedback. *British Medical Journal.* 1999 June; **318**(2).

69. Burke D, Pieterick J. *Giving Students Effective Written Feedback.* Maidenhead: Open University Press; 2010.

70. Kluger AN, Van Dijk D. Feedback, the various tasks of the doctor, and the feedforward alternative. *Medical Education.* 2010; **44**: 1166–74.

71. Nussbaum AD, Dweck CS. Defensiveness versus remediation: self-theories and modes of self-esteem maintenance. *Personality and Social Psychology Bulletin.* 2008; **34**: 599–612.

72. London Deanery. Multiprofessional faculty development: receiving feedback. [Online]; 2012. Available from: www.faculty.londondeanery.ac.uk/e-learning/feedback/receiving-feedback (accessed 24 August 2014).

73. Ashford SJ, Cummings LL. Feedback as an individual resource: personal strategies of creating information. *Organisational Behaviour and Human Performance*. 1983; **32**: 370–98.

74. Sully De Luque MF, Sommer SM. The impact of culture on feedback-seeking behaviour: an integrated model and propositions. *Academy of Management Review*. 2000 October; **25**(4): 829–49.

75. Norfolk T, Siriwardena AN. A unifying theory of clinical practice: Relationship, Diagnostics, Management and professionalism (RDM-p). *Quality in Primary Care*. 2009; 7: 37–47.

76. Eccles J, Draper J, Rutt G, *et al*. The trainee experiencing difficulty. In: *The Essential Handbook for GP Training and Education*. London: Radcliffe Publishing; 2012. pp. 446–5.

77. Jarvis P, Holford J, Griffin C. *The Theory and Practice of Learning*. 2nd ed. Abingdon: RoutledgeFalmer; 2003.

78. Mehay R, editor. *The Essential Handbook for GP Training and Education*. London: Radcliffe Publishing; 2012.

79. Middleton P, Field S. *The GP Trainers' Handbook*. Oxford: Radcliffe Medical Press; 2001.

CHAPTER 7: LEADERSHIP AND MANAGEMENT

1. Cronin C. Workplace learning: a healthcare perspective. *Education & Training*. 2014; **56**(4): 329–42.

2. Grow GO. Teaching learners to be self-directed. *Adult Education Quarterly*. 1991; **41**(3): 125–49.

3. Ham C, Hartley N. *Patient-centred Leadership: rediscovering our purpose*. London: The King's Fund; 2013. Report No.: 978 1 909029 08 8.

4. Kotter JP. *A Force for Change: how leadership differs from management*. New York, NY: The Free Press; 1990.

5. Schein EH. *Organizational Culture and Leadership*. 3rd ed. San Francisco, CA: Jossey-Bass; 2004.

6. Senge PM. *The Fifth Discipline: the art & practice of the learning organisation*. 2nd ed. London: Random House Business Books; 2006.

7. Ramsden P. *Learning to Lead in Higher Education*. London: Routledge; 1998.

8. Kotter JP. *Leading Change*. Boston, MA: Harvard Business Review Press; 2012.

9. Kübler-Ross E. *On Death and Dying*. New York, NY: Scribner; 1969.

10. Lewin K. Environmental forces in child behavior and development. In: Lewin K. *A Dynamic Theory of Personality: selected papers*. New York, NY: McGraw Hill Book Company Inc.; 1935. pp. 66–113.

11. NHS Leadership Acdemy. Leadership Framework (LF). [Online]; 2014. Available from: www.leadershipacademy.nhs.uk/discover/leadership-framework/ (accessed 29 April 2014).

12. Kouzes J, Posner B. *The Leadership Challenge: how to make extraordinary things happen in organizations*. 5th ed. San Francisco: Jossey-Bass; 2012.

13. Bass BM. *Bass & Stogdill's Handbook of Leadership: theory, research, & managerial applications*. 3rd ed. New York, NY: The Free Press; 1990.

14. Radcliffe S. *Leadership Plain and Simple*. 2nd ed. Harlow: Pearson Education Limited; 2012.

15. Goleman D, Boyatzis R, McKee A. *Primal Leadership: unleashing the power of emotional intelligence*. Boston, MA: Harvard Business Review Press; 2013.

16. Hayashi AM. When to trust your gut. *Harvard Business Review*. 2001 February: 59–65.

17. Slack N, Chambers S, Johnstone R. *Operations Management*. 6th ed. Essex: Pearson Education Limited; 2010.

18. Raven BH, French JRP Jr. Legitimate power, coercive power, and observability in social influence. *Sociometry*. 1958 June; **21**(2): 83–97.

19. Herzberg F. *Work and the Nature of Man*. Cleveland, OH: The World Publishing Company; 1966.

20. Dweck CS, Leggett EL. A social-cognitive approach to motivation and personality. *Psychological Review*. 1988; **95**(2): 256–73.

21. Brewster C, Fager J. *Increasing Student Engagement and Motivation: from time-on-task to homework*. North West Regional Educational Laboratory; 2000.

22. Goldman S. The Educational Kanban: promoting effective self-directed adult learning in medical education. *Academic Medicine*. 2009 July; **84**(7): 927–34.

23. De Bono E. *Six Thinking Hats*. London: Penguin Books Ltd.; 2000.

CHAPTER 8: SUMMARY

1. Barr H, Helme M, D'Avray L. *Occasional Paper No 12: developing interprofessional education in health and social care courses in the United Kingdom*. Health Sciences and Practice Subject Centre, Higher Education Academy. 2011 September. Available at: www.health.heacademy. ac.uk/lenses/occasionalpapers/m10247.html (accessed 22 August 2014).

Index

CPD with Radcliffe

You can now use a selection of our books to achieve CPD (Continuing Professional Development) points through directed reading.

We provide a free online form and downloadable certificate for your appraisal portfolio. Look for the CPD logo and register with us at: www.radcliffehealth.com/cpd

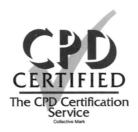